Intraocular Surgery

Thomas H. Williamson

Intraocular Surgery

A Basic Surgical Guide

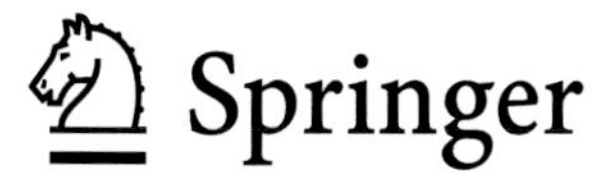

Thomas H. Williamson
Department of Ophthalmology
St Thomas Hospital
London
UK

ISBN 978-3-319-27988-6 ISBN 978-3-319-27990-9 (eBook)
DOI 10.1007/978-3-319-27990-9

Library of Congress Control Number: 2016934931

Springer Cham Heidelberg New York Dordrecht London

Printed on acid-free paper

Springer International Publishing AG Switzerland is part of Springer Science+Business Media (www.springer.com)

Preface

For the majority, the most exciting and challenging aspect of ophthalmology is surgery. However we often start our training in the specialty without any surgical grounding, immediately or rapidly entering the operating room and commencing surgery. This book is an attempt to provide some of the basic information that you require to perform maximally in this complex and intricate surgery, thereby giving the reader a head start.

The descriptions in this book are intended to provide the reader with all sorts of insights and information to allow the development of a thoughtful and considered approach to surgery. Some of the information will be obvious to some but not to others. The processes should make you scrutinize with more intelligence the surgical methods you are employing.

This is a text of basic principles and methods and has been written to allow easy communication and assimilation of the information. Detailed descriptions of particular surgical operations have been avoided as the aim is to inform the reader of the basics, which will be relevant to many different operations. It is often failure to understand the simple basics, which hampers progress. Hopefully, the simple steps of surgery can be performed to a much higher standard after reading this book, improving the quality of the surgery overall.

Finally to take the readers' interpretation of surgery to a new level, we have introduced some examinations by finite element analysis. This reverse engineering method allows an investigator the opportunity to more fully understand their craft. Throughout this book, you will see thought-provoking examples of the application of this method used as a stimulant for further analysis and investigation of the subject of ophthalmic surgery.

London, UK Thomas H. Williamson

Contents

1 Surgical Philosophy 1
Achieving Your Objective 1
Margin of Safety 2
Risks and Benefits 2
Changing Methods 2
Complications 5
Surgical Drift 6
The Pareto Principle 6
Reducing the Chance of Error 7
Simplify 7
Compartmentalize 7
The Early Majority 7
Finally 7

2 Finite Element Analysis (FEA), Material Properties and Tissue Geometry in Ophthalmology 9
Introduction 9
Material Properties 10
Young's Modulus of Elasticity and Yield Strength 10
Bulk Modulus 12
Shear Modulus 12
Poisson Ratio 13
Density 13
Tissue Geometry 15
Meshing of the Model 16
Finite Element Analysis 16
Analogies in Science Communication 17
References 18

3 Surgical Principles: Instruments 21
Introduction. 21
Forceps 21
Visualisation 27
Mobile Tissue 27
Closure Mechanisms. 27
Angulation. 28

4 Surgical Principles: Wounds and Tissue Manipulation 39
Incisions 39
FEA, Appreciation of the Surgical Planes in Microsurgery 49
Corneal Section and the Surgical Plane 49
Rigid and Malleable 49
Scissors 50
Lamellar Wounds 51
Curved Wounds. 52
FEA. 57
FEA, Continuous Curvilinear Capsulorhexis and the Surgical Plane. . . . 62
Finite Element Analysis Application of Young's Modulus in Ophthalmic Surgery 68
FEA Continuous Circular Capsulorhexis and Capsular Fold Configurations 70
Zero Fold Configuration 71
Single Fold Configuration. 72
Double Fold Configuration 73
FEA Capsulorhexis Size and Nucleus Rotation 73
FEA Capsulorhexis Size and Nucleus Cracking. 76
FEA Sculpting Central Groove and the Surgical Plane 76
FEA Rotation of the Nucleus and the Surgical Plane. 78
FEA Cracking the Nucleus into Quadrants and the Surgical Plane . . . 78
References. 86

5 Compartments. 87
FEA Pressure Balance on Both Sides. 87
FEA Choroidal Haemorrhage. 92
Arc of Safety. 95
FEA Zonular Support 100
References. 110

6 Machines 111
Pumps 114
Phacoemulsification 116
Guillotine 116
FEA Ultrasonic Phacoemulsification 118
Duty Cycle 123
References. 123

7 Fluids ... 125
Flow ... 125
Viscosity ... 127
Viscoelastic Fluids ... 127
Diffusion and Convection ... 130
Convection ... 131
Interfacial Tension ... 132
Emulsion ... 132
Evaporation ... 132
Gases ... 133

8 Microscopes, Light and Lasers ... 135
Field of View and Magnification ... 135
Fibre Optics ... 136
Laser ... 136
Yag Laser ... 141

9 Suturing ... 143
Single Sutures ... 144
Continuous Sutures ... 148
Knots ... 154

Index ... 165

Chapter 1
Surgical Philosophy

Before embarking on surgery at the surgeon needs to have a clear approach to the principles of achieving high success. This will include a continuous monitoring and assessment of surgical methods and clinical outcomes. There are certain principles that the surgeon must be aware of.

Two major principles are:

1. achieving your objective
2. maintaining a margin of safety

Achieving Your Objective

It is important that the surgeon has a clear idea about what outcome is being achieved through surgery. That outcome must always relate to the patient's well being and not just to the surgical challenge ahead.

Although surgery is a technical exercise, the satisfaction of achieving a good technical outcome is overridden by the need to improve or protect the patient's quality of life. The surgeon can enjoy the technical challenge, application of surgical skills, and the perfect anatomical outcome but all of these are useless if there is no clinical benefit.

The surgeon will need to obtain many capabilities to achieve the objective, including knowledge, experience, empathy, manual dexterity and surgical skills. It will be a lifelong exercise trying to maximise all of these.

T.H. Williamson, *Intraocular Surgery: A Basic Surgical Guide*,
DOI 10.1007/978-3-319-27990-9_1

Margin of Safety

It is possible to have an operation which can achieve an outcome but is too dangerous to perform. For this reason the surgeon must always factor in the margin of safety for each step in a procedure or for the procedure itself in total. A high margin of safety is likely to improve the capability to achieve an objective. However there comes point where, if the surgeon only considers the margin of safety and is too cautious in the approach to surgery, this will have a detrimental effect on achieving objectives. For example, a surgeon may perform an operation on the heart to minimise the chance of mortality, by only performing minimal and safe surgery. Being too cautious and unambitious in the surgical procedure may leave the patient with increased morbidity from continuing cardiac disorder. Therefore too much caution and safety can lead to a less effective outcome (Fig. 1.1).

Risks and Benefits

Another way to look at this is to look at the risks and benefits of a surgical procedure or indeed of any steps in that procedure. There is a balance between the risks of doing something and the benefits obtained. In simple terms the benefits should outweigh the risks. This may not always be easily determined however. A surgeon may feel the need to add a surgical step to an existing procedure. There may or may not be enough information available to decide whether the risks outweigh the benefits or vice versa. It may take time for the 2 parameters to be understood through the experience of employing the extra surgical step or from the experience of others. In general however it is beholden on the surgeon to make some assessment prior to adopting a change (Figs. 1.2, 1.3, and 1.4).

Changing Methods

One of the great things about surgery is the constant change in methodology. An up-to-date Surgeon will be confronted by many changes in surgical procedures in their working life. Changing what you trust and understand is not always easy to do.

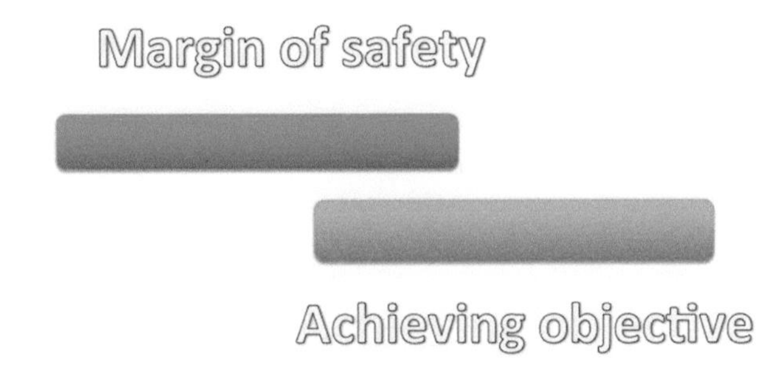

Fig. 1.1 Care must be taken to stay within the margin of safety when trying to achieve your goal

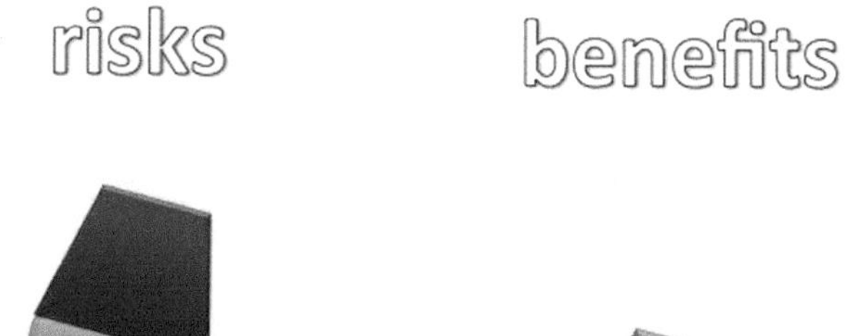

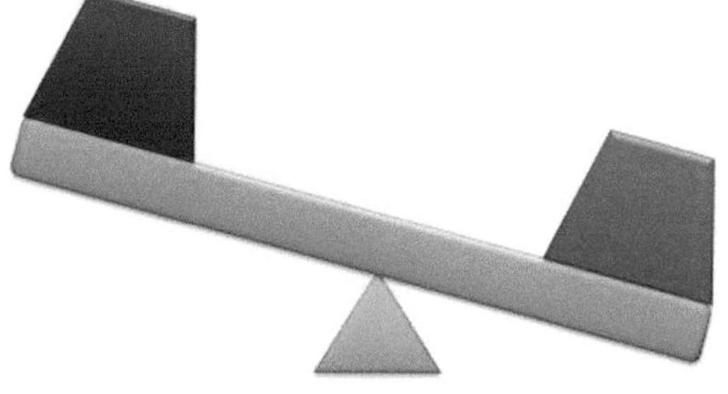

Fig. 1.2 There is a balance to be found between risks and benefits

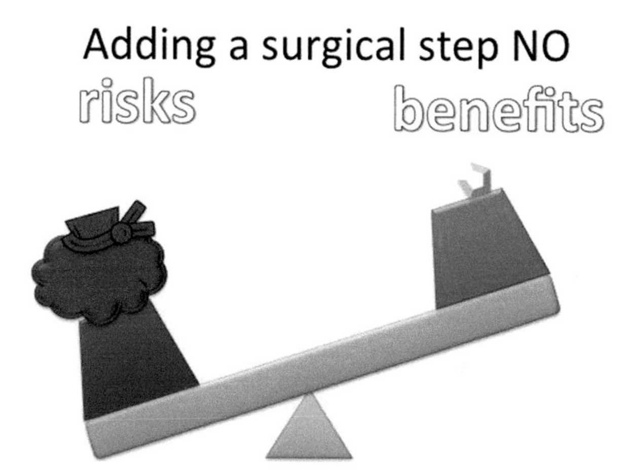

Fig. 1.3 Sometimes the risks outweigh the benefits

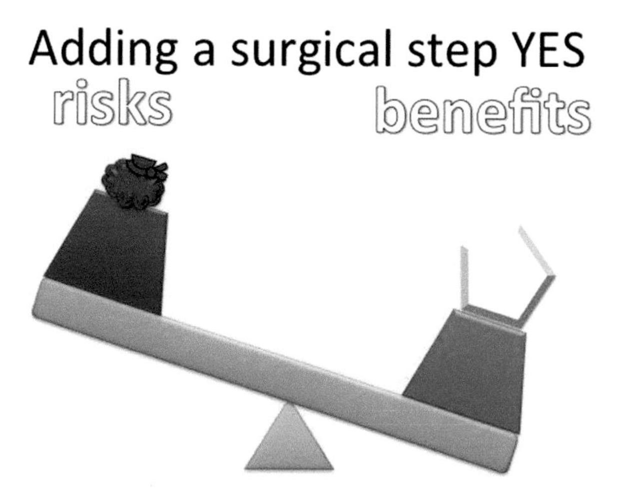

Fig. 1.4 The benefits may outweigh the risks

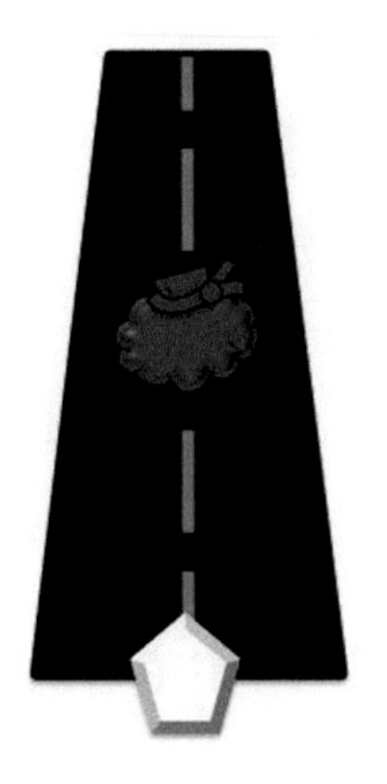

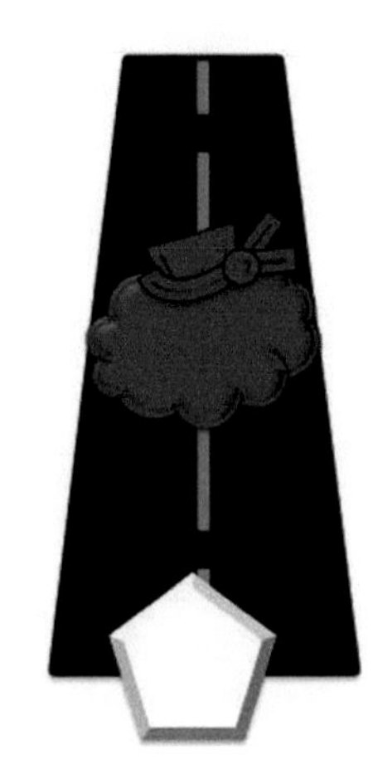

Fig. 1.5 When changing routes to your goal try to decide if the "bag" of risks are too great or if the objective provides enough extra benefit

Sticking with an old method has the comfort of the knowledge that experience has brought, and safety margins are likely to be at their maximum for that procedure. In time however, complacency can creep in which can prevent the surgeon moving on to a better modern procedure or even create inattention to detail for the existing method (Fig. 1.5).

Moving to a new method can provide the stimulation of a new challenge. Lack of experience of a new procedure usually increases risk of complications at least in the short-term. There may also be unforeseen consequences that must be watched for.

Again when changing method the surgeon must assess how large the potential benefit is and balance this with the potential for risks on the way to the change. If the risks are very large for a small benefit or the risks are very small for a large benefit then the decision to change is easy. However, the risks maybe small with a small benefit or the risks may be a large with a large potential benefit, in which case the decision to change is much more complex and must be related to how much the patient needs the extra benefit (Fig. 1.6).

A figure can be drawn of the proportion of people who fall into the groups

Innovators
Early adopters
Early majority
Late majority
Laggards

It is likely that the surgeons who fall into the group "early majority" will most safely operate upon the patient. The innovators and early adopters may put the patient at higher risk by taking on a new method before experience has been gained about it risk profile. The late majority and laggards are too slow to provide the benefits of a new technique to the patients (Fig. 1.7).

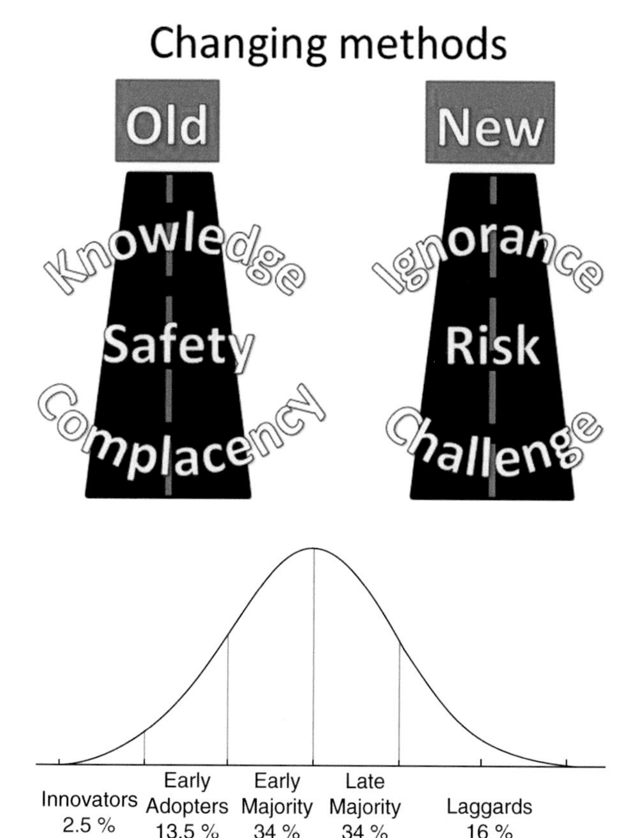

Fig. 1.6 Consider these factors when you are thinking about making a change

Fig. 1.7 There are surgeons with different approaches to change. Perhaps the the most effective group to be in and safest for your patients is the early majority grouping

Complications

Any surgeon who claims never to have complications is deluded, dishonest or unable to diagnose error. There is a random element to our interaction with biological tissue which cannot be completely controlled for. The complex relationship of genetics and environment on human tissue is such that all tissues will have variability from patient to patient. How a tissue handles or reacts to what we do to it will become familiar with experience within certain boundaries, however surprises are never far away. What surgeons do is inherently dangerous to that part of the body under operation. It is worth remembering that we only have approximately 100 years experience of surgery of any sophistication on the eye.

It is a fact of life that complications will happen. The surgeon strives to minimise risk. The perfect procedure avoids complications but this procedure probably does not exist. Our endpoint is a successful outcome, certainly the avoidance of complications helps achieve this outcome. If complications occur then it is important that the surgeon is equipped to manage them. Often managing the complication successfully, will achieve the desired outcome: surgery fails when there is inability to manage the complication.

Surgical Drift

Be aware that when a surgeon has great familiarity with a procedure and comfort with it, that this can, in fact, lead to error. Often the use of a methodology is not a choice of "yes" or "no". Instead there is a spectrum of its usage, for example, using a very small wound to do an operation can vary from very small to extremely small. Sometimes the surgeon may feel that by making the wound smaller and smaller he is performing a better operation. I see this like a sailor who has become comfortable bobbing along in the wind and has forgotten that he may be heading for an underwater reef and disaster. The surgeon may perform a procedure with a smaller and smaller wound. Gradually over time the wound is reducing in size, perhaps for a cosmetic reason or other functional reason. However there may be a threshold size of the wound where other problems appear, for example limiting the exposure of the surgical area causes failure to see and remove a tumour completely. In ophthalmology you might gradually increase the sclerotomy of a trabeculectomy to maximize the drop in IOP but soon start to see patients with hypotony and choroidal effusion. Therefore even though you have used a surgical method for a long time it is worth reconsidering each step and re-balancing it for risk and benefit (Fig. 1.8).

The Pareto Principle

This principle also known as the 80–20 rule is a truism, which is worth remembering. Essentially, to achieve a certain outcome you can consider that 80 % of the effect comes from 20 % of the input. It is much harder to achieve the next 20 % of

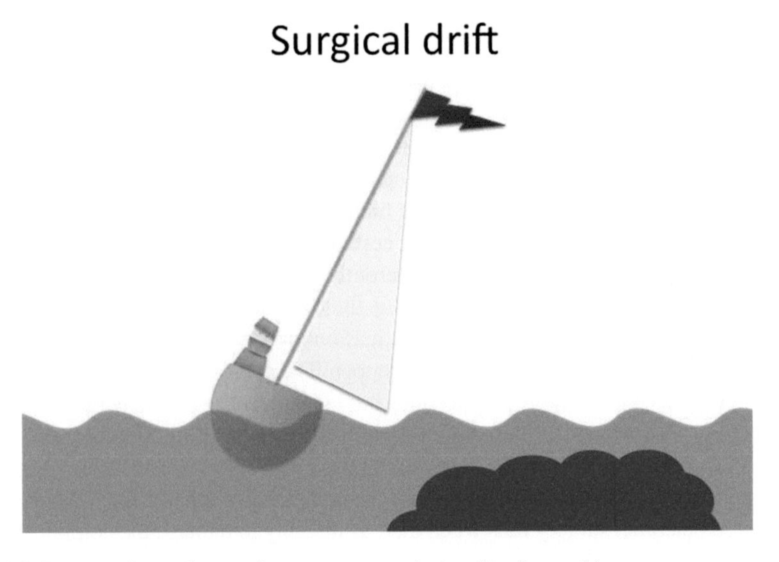

Fig. 1.8 Beware of complacency because you may be heading for trouble

the effect. For example in retinal detachment surgery, with large mixed presentations, it has been routine to achieve success rates around 85 %. However it has been extremely difficult, despite great effort, to push that success rate to 90 % or more.

Reducing the Chance of Error

Some simple rules, which are applicable to all surgeries may help you reduce error.

Simplify

If you can take 1 step to achieve an outcome this is usually better than taking 2 because the second step will bring with it a collection of complications. Unless you can convince yourself that those complications significantly improve the benefit the second step is best left alone.

Compartmentalize

For complex surgery it is usually possible to break the operation down into compartments. Each of those compartments may be very familiar. An example would be the combination of the vitrectomy and cataract surgery. By performing the whole cataract operation to its completion and then the vitrectomy afterwards both operations can be performed in a familiar way reducing the opportunity for error.

The Early Majority

If you want to be kind to your patients let others do the testing of innovation on their patients and wait before implementing the changes on yours. However be aware that surgical innovations can improve outcomes and adopt the good ones early to the benefit of your patients.

Finally

Remember neither success nor failure is all about you alone. The environment in which you work restricts or enhances your ability to perform at the highest level.

The whole system contributes to your performance and there will be areas, which you cannot improve. The Japanese call it Kaisen (improvement) when they need to change something for the better but not all systems are responsive to this.

The organization within which you work must provide the opportunity for you to suggest change, be responsive to that request and be able to implement. This is not always the case and it is not your responsibility to carry the blame for failure for areas within which you cannot influence improvement.

Chapter 2
Finite Element Analysis (FEA), Material Properties and Tissue Geometry in Ophthalmology

Introduction

Ophthalmologists deal with solid tissues such as cornea, sclera, retina, choroid, iris, crystalline lens, nerve, muscle, fat and bone and also with fluids such as aqueous humour, and blood. Solid and liquid materials have inherent physical properties related to their components like elasticity, viscosity and density. Such properties determine the materials' interaction and behaviour. Computation of the extent of displacement, deformation and strain caused by shear, compressive, or tensile forces on materials of inherent properties and simple dimensions like squares or circles can be achieved through simple mathematical computations. The computation, however, becomes complicated when the dimensions as well as the properties of the material are more complex. Therefore for complex problems, the science of finite element analysis is used. Finite element analysis exploits material properties and dimensions to solve complex problems in the universe using mathematical approaches [1]. Finite element analysis divides complex dimensions into smaller squares, triangles or hexagons to build finite element models that could be analysed using numerical methods. Finite element analysis also allows detailed visualisation of where the structure bends or twists, and indicates the distribution of stresses and displacements. In ophthalmology, this science has helped in the provision of mathematical solutions to surgical and biological problems and to predict the optimum surgical manoeuvres to achieve certain goals [2]. In this section we will describe the basics of finite element method and its applications in ophthalmology.

T.H. Williamson, *Intraocular Surgery: A Basic Surgical Guide*,
DOI 10.1007/978-3-319-27990-9_2

Material Properties

Application of force on materials leads to a change in the geometry of the material. The force used is called "stress" and presented as force per unit area and the resultant deformation in the material is called "strain". Strain is proportional to the stress up to a limit and is dependent on the material properties. Therefore, material properties need to be known to replicate the original material onto the computer and achieve stress-strain analysis. The basic material properties that need to be known for accurate finite element analysis are:

- Young's modulus of elasticity and yield strength
- Bulk and shear modulus
- Poisson's ratio
- Density.

It must be noted that a wide range of material property values for ocular tissues have been reported in the literature, therefore the values need to be considered carefully when used in analysis to avoid inaccuracies. Authors of this book and authors of previous finite element analysis studies have found the data in Table 2.1 most reliable (Fig. 2.1).

Young's Modulus of Elasticity and Yield Strength

Young's modulus is the force (per unit area) that is needed to stretch (or compress) a material sample. Elasticity is the ability of a material to return to its previous state after the applied stress is removed. If the amount of strain produced in the material is directly proportional to the stress applied on the material, such materials are called linearly elastic materials where stress applied is uniformly spread all throughout the body of the material. For such types of material the stress-strain relationship is linear as it is shown in (Fig. 2.1) [16, 17].

Young's modulus is used to determine stress–a strain relationship in a linearly elastic portion of a stress-strain curve and is always below the yield point, beyond which the material starts to deform. Most of the linearly elastic materials retain some amount of deformation even after the stress applied is removed. This is called the plasticity of the material. If the stress applied is still not removed, the material completely deforms or it completely fails to regain its previous shape. This point is called failure. A yield strength or yield point is the minimum amount of stress (force/unit area) required for the permanent deformation (failure) of a material (example, fracture of bone).

If this failure occurs because of compressive or tensile stresses applied, then it is called compressive or tensile failure, respectively. Imagine pulling a rubber band where it first gets stretched (elasticity), then slightly loses its shape beyond the yield point (plastic deformation) and finally breaks at the point of failure. In case of brittle

Table 2.1 Shows some of the known material properties, a wide range of values has been reported in the literature, and therefore the values need to be considered carefully when used in analysis to avoid inaccuracies

Tissue	Young's modulus MPa	Shear modulus MPa	Poisson ratio	Bulk	Density kg/m^3	References
Six muscles Linear elastic	11.0000	3.9286	0.4000	18.3333	1600.0000	[3]
Ciliary body Linear elastic	11.0000	3.9286	0.4000	18.3333	1600.0000	[3]
Eyeball	0.5000	0.1786	0.4000	0.8333		[4]
Skin	1.0000	0.3448	0.4500	3.3333		[5]
Sclera	5.5000	0.0103	0.4540	0.1087	1200.0000	[5, 6]
Nerve	5.5000	1.8707	0.4700	30.5556		[5]
Fatty tissue Linear elastic	0.0470	0.0158	0.4900	0.7833	999.0000	[3]
Vitreous Linear elastic	0.0420	0.0141	0.4900	0.7000	999.0000	[3]
Aqueous Linear elastic	0.0370	0.0124	0.4900	0.6167	999.0000	[3]
Cornea	4.9611	1.6600	0.4943	145.0000	1149.0000	[5, 6]
Lamina Cribrosa	0.3000	0.1001	0.4990	50.0000		[5]
Retina	0.0300	0.0101	0.4900	0.5000	1100.0000	[6] [2]
Young Person Capsule	0.7000	0.2381	0.4700	3.8889		[7, 8]
Old person Capsule and ILM	2.1000	0.7143	0.4700	11.6667		[7–9]
Zonule	1.5000	0.5102	0.4700	8.3333		[7, 10, 11]
Young Person Lens	2.0600	0.0000	0.4700	11.4444	1100.0000	[10, 12, 13]
Old person lens	6.8900	0.0000	0.4700	38.2778		[10, 12, 13]
Choroid	0.0652					[14]
Bone trabecular tissue from the femoral neck	6900		0.3000			[15]
Bone interstitial tissue from the diaphyseal cortex	25,000	9615.385	0.3000	20833.3		[15]

Authors of this book and authors of previous finite element analysis studies have found the data in this table most reliable

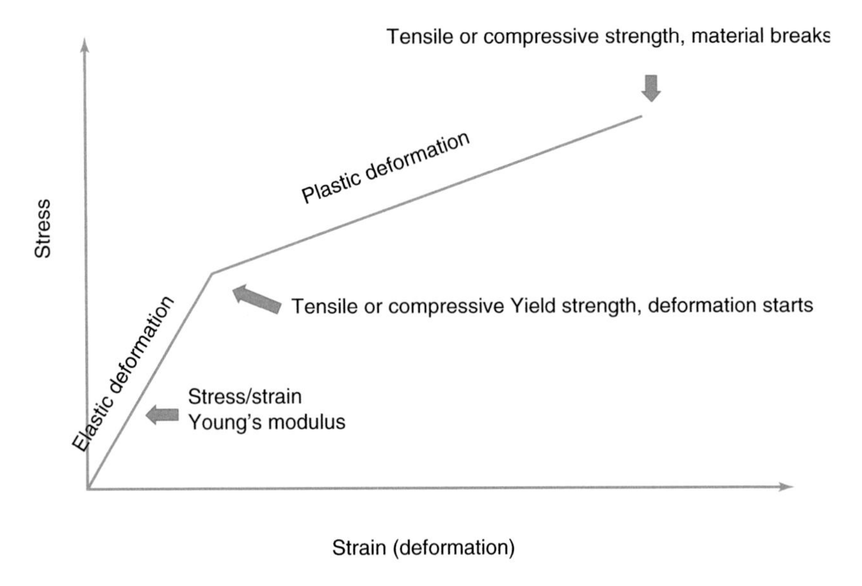

Fig. 2.1 The stress/strain relationship

materials, the material, beyond the yield point, directly undergoes failure (breaks) without going through a phase of plastic deformation [18].

Application of Young's Modulus in Ophthalmic Surgery

See Chap. 4 for some examples.

Bulk Modulus

Bulk modulus describes the material's response (resistance) to uniform pressure. The response of a cricket/tennis/rubber ball getting compressed uniformly from all directions (when squeezing) is described by the Bulk modulus of the material of cricket/tennis/rubber ball [19]. Sclera inherently has lower bulk modulus compared with bone; therefore the magnitude of the total deformation in the sclera is more than the bone when pressure is applied uniformly in all directions (Fig. 2.2).

Shear Modulus

Shear modulus quantifies the material's response to shearing strain and is concerned with the deformation of a solid when it experiences a force parallel to one of its surfaces, while its opposite face experiences an opposing force (friction).

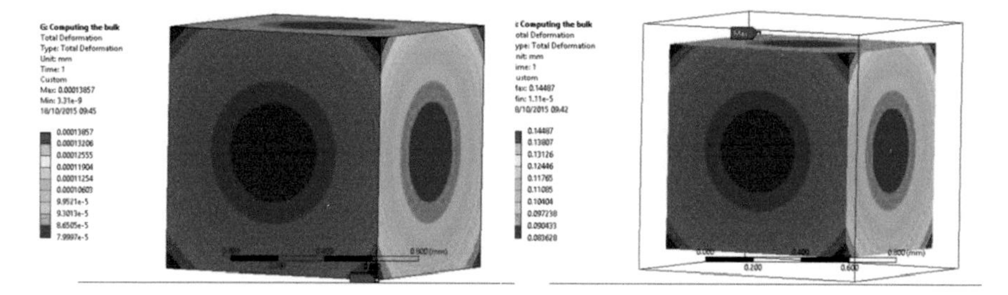

Fig. 2.2 FEA shows the effect of the 10 N pressure applied uniformly from all 6 directions on 1 mm3 of tissue. Left shows the tissues with material properties similar to bone showing minimal deformation. Right shows the tissue with material properties similar to sclera showing more deformation

Imagine peeling an epiretinal membrane off the surface of the retina by folding it on itself and pulling it backward. This manoeuvre will result in tension in the membrane and shear at the pegs that connect the epiretinal membrane to the retina. Using finite element analysis you can compute the magnitude of shear stress generated during pulling the epiretinal membranes. See Chap. 3.

Poisson Ratio

When a material is compressed in one direction, it usually tends to expand in the other two directions perpendicular to the direction of compression and vice versa. This is called Poisson effect [20]. Poisson ratio is the ratio of the relative contraction strain (transverse strain) perpendicular to the applied load to relative extension strain (axial strain) parallel to applied load. When the eyeball is hit with a tennis ball approaching in a direction parallel to its axis, it tends to expand in its radial axis. The magnitude of the radial deformation is dependent on the eyeball's Poisson ratio, and because of the geometry of the eye this maximum deformation tends to occur at the limbal area. This explains why sometimes the iris, cilliary body, zonular and/or retinal dialysis can happen after blunt traumas, in addition to rupture of the sclera at the cornea-scleral limbus (Figs. 2.3 and 2.4).

Density

Density of a material is basically an indication of compactness of a material based on how dense its micro structural arrangement is at a molecular level (Fig. 2.5). This is the basic need for assessment of the strength of a material which directly or indirectly affects all other material properties. All biological tissue is neither homogeneous nor isotropic, therefore their physical properties vary both in location and in direction [1].

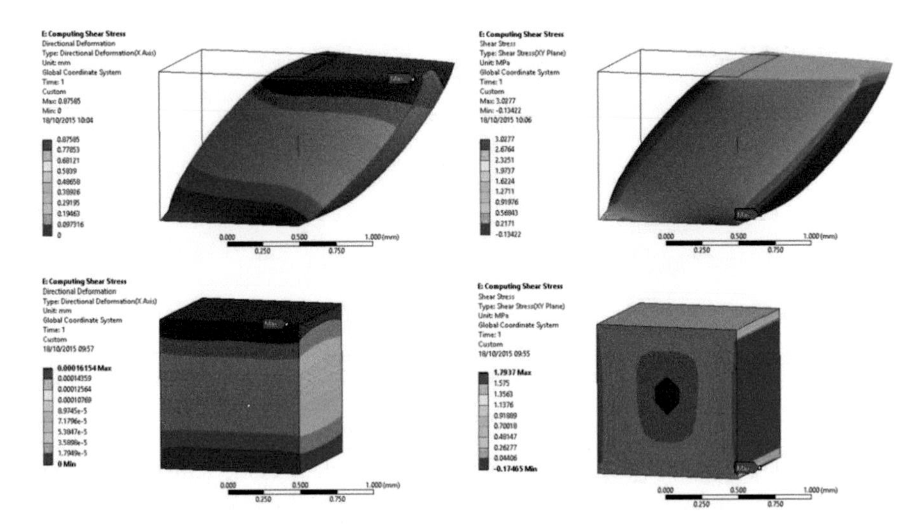

Fig. 2.3 FEA shows the effect of 1 N shear shower force applied on the top surface of a 1 mm^3 tissue. The top row shows the deformation and the shear stress in a tissue with material properties similar to that of the cornea; and the bottom row shows the deformation and the shear stress in a tissue with material properties similar to that of the bone

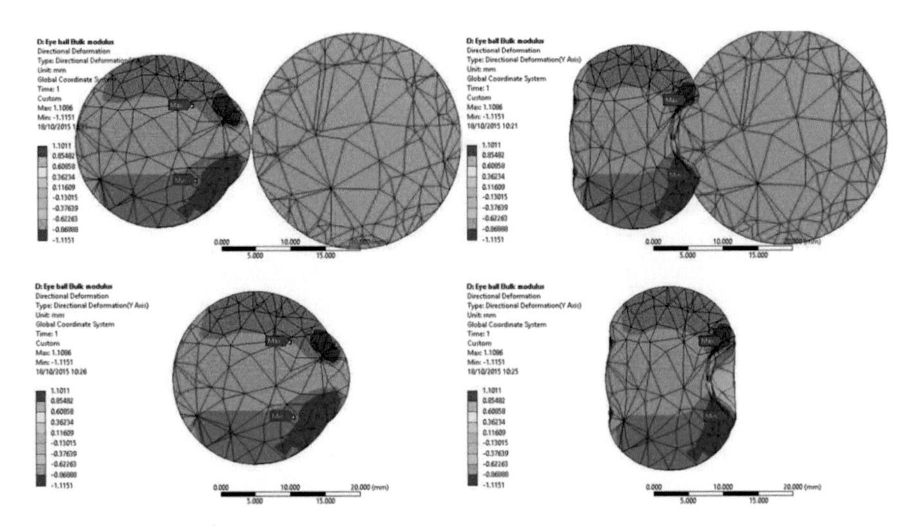

Fig. 2.4 Shows an eyeball being hit by a tennis ball in its axial direction. The maximum radial deformation generated is located at the limbus. Top left shows the eyeball and the tennis ball just before the impact; top right shows the eyeball and the tennis ball during the impact; bottom left shows the eyeball only, just before the impact; bottom left shows the eyeball only, during the impact

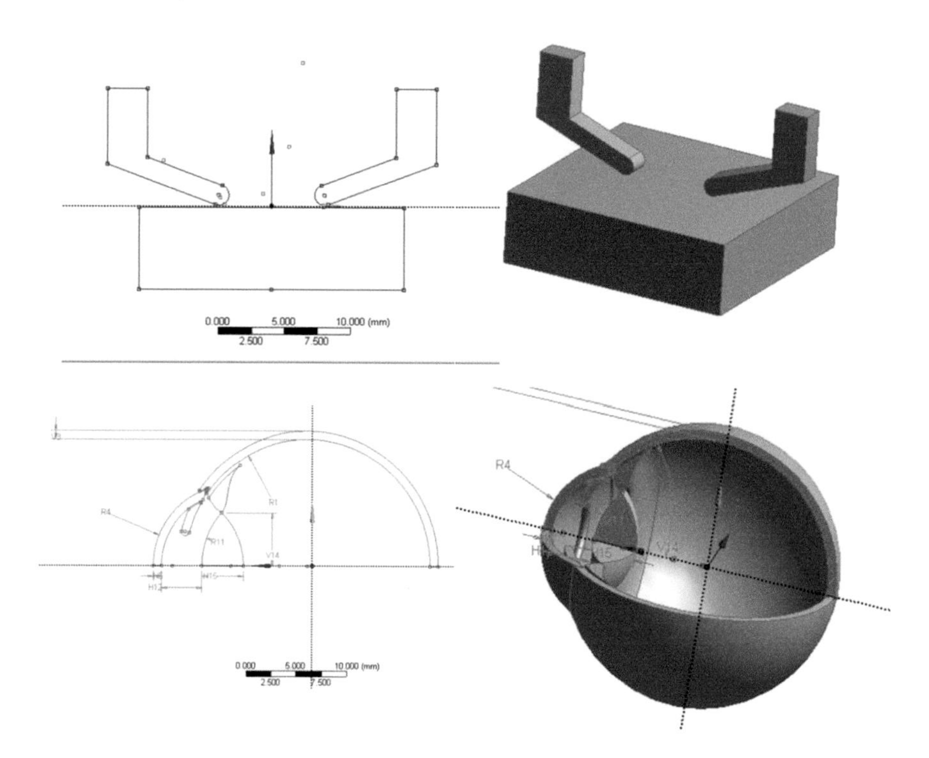

Fig. 2.5 Shows examples of Extrude and Revolve techniques to create solid parts by sketching the shape on an existing planar surface. Top row is an extruded feature

Tissue Geometry

Geometries, dimensions and inter point measurements are essential for precise modelling of biological tissues, they could be obtained from CT scan studies of the areas of interest. Some commercially available software is capable of generating meshed 3D models directly from CT scan images. However generic anatomical dimensions are commonly used for ophthalmology research purposes. Using general values helps to create cleaner geometrical models that would take less time in computing compared to models created from scanned data that usually embrace artefacts. Table 2.2 shows some generic geometrical values of the ocular tissues.

Geometrical dimensions could then be transformed into solid features using a variety of techniques. The most common techniques to create solid features are Extrude and Revolve. These techniques create features by sketching the shape on an existing planar surface, the extruded features are then created ‘normal’ to the sketch plane and revolved features are revolved about a sketched centreline. Examples of Extrude and Revolve features are shown in the figure (Fig. 2.5).

Table 2.2 Shows generic dimensions of the ocular tissues used in previous finite elements analysis studies

Name coded name	Baseline	Units	Source
Internal radius of eye shell	12.0	mm	[21]
Scleral thickness at canal	0.4	mm	[21]
Laminar thickness at axis	0.3	mm	[21]
Retinal thickness	0.2	mm	[21]
Scleral shell thickness	0.8	mm	[21]
Lamina Cribrosa anterior surface radius	0.95	mm	[21]
Pia mater thickness	0.06	mm	[21]
Laminar curvature	0.2	mm	[21]
Canal wall angle to the horizontal	60	deg	[21]
ILM thickness	2.5	micron	[22]
ERM thickness	20	micron	[2]

Meshing of the Model

This model is then meshed using finite element software to cut the model into a finite number of smaller sections called elements. The meshed element is called finite element model, with each element having properties exactly as the original material. The accuracy of the final results of the analysis depends on the type and the number of the elements. Figure 2.6 shows the previous solid featured 3D models being divided into simpler dimensions [23].

Finite Element Analysis

The natural physical conditions such as force or temperature around the original object (tissue/metal) are applied on the finite number of elements of the finite element model using various software programs. The software carries out structural analysis that comprises of a set of physical laws and mathematics required to analyse and predict the behaviour of structures, the integrity of which is judged largely by their ability to withstand loads.

Finally the results are computed to show the outcome in terms of deformation and strain. Hence finite element analysis is basically a reconstruction of stress, strain, and deformation in digital structure.

Finite element analysis is commonly used to help in constructing buildings, bridges, aircraft, ships, and cars. In medicine, structural analysis incorporates the fields of mechanics and dynamics to analyse biological tissues. From a theoretical perspective the primary goal of structural analysis is the computation of deformations, internal forces and stresses. In practice, structural analysis can be viewed more abstractly as a method to prove the soundness of a design without a

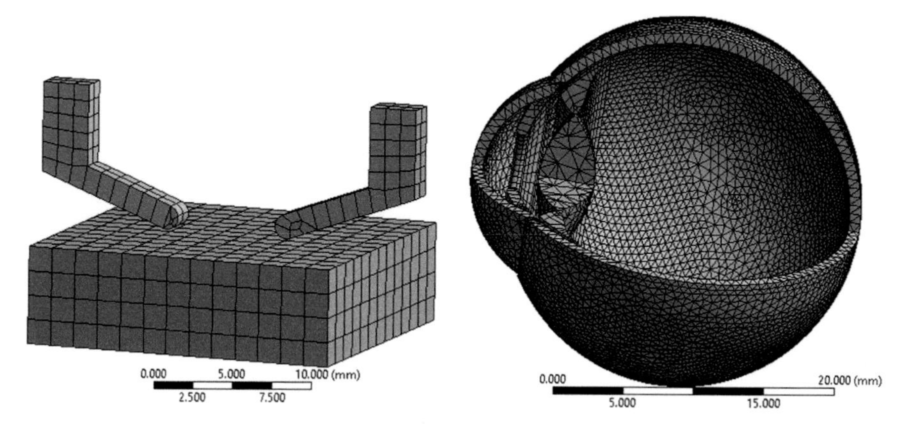

Fig. 2.6 Shows complex 3D models divided into simpler dimensions using software. Each meshed model consists of a varying number of nodes depending on the shape of the element triangle/hexagon). Left shows forceps grasping tip over a tissue. Right shows a meshed eyeball model

dependence on directly testing it. The finite element approach of structural analysis is an advanced matrix algebraic method to model an entire structure with one-, two-, and three-dimensional elements [23].

Analogies in Science Communication

Peter Atkins, in his book "Creation Revisited", uses personification analogy when considering the refraction of a light beam, passing into a medium of higher refractive index, which slows it down. The beam behaves as if trying to minimize the time taken to travel to an end point. Atkins imagines it as a lifeguard on a beach racing to rescue a drowning swimmer. Should he head straight for the swimmer? No, because he can run faster than he can swim and would be wise to increase the dry-land proportion of his travel time. Should he run to a point on the beach directly opposite his target, thereby minimizing his swimming time? Better, but still not the best. Calculation (if he had time to do it) would disclose to the lifeguard an optimum intermediate angle, yielding the ideal combination of fast running followed by inevitably slower swimming. Atkins concluded that this is exactly the behaviour of light passing into a denser medium. But how does light know, apparently in advance, which is the briefest path? And, anyway, why should it care? Atkins develops these questions in a fascinating exposition, inspired by quantum theory. Richard Dawkins, in his book "The Selfish Gene" states that analogies of this kind are not just a quaint didactic device. They can also help a professional scientist to get the right answer, in the face of tricky temptations to error where it is very easy to get the wrong answer.

Sophisticated ophthalmic machines are based on established laws of physics to achieve certain goals. Most trainee ophthalmologists usually have no previous experience with such devices, teaching trainees the relevant laws of physics per se would enhance the depth and the breadth of their theoretical knowledge but will not greatly help with their surgical experience. On the other hand careful and cautious use of analogies to simulate some of the surgical events to actions familiar to the trainees, often turns out to be the shortest route to rescuing a trainee surgeon drowning in muddle.

References

1. Sundar SS, et al. Finite element analysis: a maxillofacial surgeon's perspective. J Maxillofac Oral Surg. 2012;11(2):206–11.
2. Dogramaci M, Williamson TH. Dynamics of epiretinal membrane removal off the retinal surface: a computer simulation project. Br J Ophthalmol. 2013;97(9):1202–7.
3. Power ED. A nonlinear finite element model of the human eye to investigate ocular injuries from night vision goggles. Thesis submitted to Virginia Polytechnic Institute and State University; Virginia: Blacksburg; 2001.
4. Schutte S, et al. A finite-element analysis model of orbital biomechanics. Vision Res. 2006;46(11):1724–31.
5. Cirovic S, et al. Computer modelling study of the mechanism of optic nerve injury in blunt trauma. Br J Ophthalmol. 2006;90(6):778–83.
6. Rossi T, et al. Primary blast injury to the eye and orbit: finite element modeling. Invest Ophthalmol Visual Sci. 2012;53(13):8057–66.
7. Wilde GS. Measurement of human lens stiffness for modelling presbyopia treatments. Oxford: Oxford University; 2011.
8. Fisher R. Elastic constants of the human lens capsule. J Physiol. 1969;201(1):1–19.
9. Halfter W, et al. Protein composition and biomechanical properties of in vivo-derived basement membranes. Cell Adh Migr. 2013;7(1):64–71.
10. Stitzel JD, et al. Blunt trauma of the aging eye: injury mechanisms and increasing lens stiffness. Arch Ophthalmol. 2005;123(6):789–94.
11. Schachar RA, et al. The relationship between accommodative amplitude and the ratio of central lens thickness to its equatorial diameter in vertebrate eyes. Br J Ophthalmol. 2007;91(6):812–7.
12. Schachar RA. The mechanism of accommodation and presbyopia. Int Ophthalmol Clin. 2006;46(3):39–61.
13. Hermans E, et al. Change in the accommodative force on the lens of the human eye with age. Vision Res. 2008;48(1):119–26.
14. Wu W, Peters W, Hammer ME. Basic mechanical properties of retina in simple elongation. J Biomech Eng. 1987;109(1):65–7.
15. Zysset PK, et al. Elastic modulus and hardness of cortical and trabecular bone lamellae measured by nanoindentation in the human femur. J Biomech. 1999;32(10):1005–12.
16. Truesdell C. Rational mechanics. New York: Academic Press; 1983.
17. Huston RL. Principles of biomechanics. Washington, DC: CRC Press; 2009.
18. Flinn RA, Trojan PK. Engineering materials and their applications. Engineering materials and their applications, 4th ed, by Richard A. Flinn, Paul K. Trojan, pp. 1056. ISBN 0-471-12508-3. Wiley-VCH, December 1994. 1.

19. Nave,C. Hyperphysics–bulk elastic properties. 2014, Georgia State University, Department of Physics and Astronomy. Available from internet: http://hyperphysicsphyastr.gsu.edu/hbase/permot3.html.
20. Gercek H. Poisson's ratio values for rocks. Int J Rock Mech Min Sci. 2007;44(1):1–13.
21. Sigal IA, Flanagan JG, Ethier CR. Factors influencing optic nerve head biomechanics. Invest Ophthalmol Vis Sci. 2005;46(11):4189.
22. Foos RY. Vitreoretinal juncture; topographical variations. Invest Ophthalmol. 1972;11(10):801–8.
23. Bhavikatti S. Finite element analysis. New Delhi: New Age International; 2005.

Chapter 3
Surgical Principles: Instruments

Introduction

Before starting surgery it is worth considering instrumentation and how it works. Surgeons will more effectively employ the instruments if they have good insights into their function.

Issues to consider

- Application of forces
- Contact area
- Dynamic interaction
- Visualization of the contact area

Forceps

Consider the "toothed" forceps. This is an instrument used primarily to grasp rigid tissue. A typical design involves interlocking teeth, which come together when the surgeon applies pressure thereby apposing the shafts of the handle. The teeth are not angled at 90° to the shafts because the tip of the forceps would not be presented to the tissue. Instead the teeth are angled 45° or 60°, for example, so that once the tooth has engaged the tissue with further pressure on the handle the natural movement of the teeth is into the tissue. In this way the teeth are inserted into the surface of the tissue. This creates a minute area of damage to the tissue, but ensures a good grip (Figs. 3.1, 3.2, and 3.3).

Another function of instrumentation may be to lift an object off a surface, for example grasping a strand of a suture, which is lying on the conjunctiva. In this circumstance the desire is not to injure the underlying tissue or indeed to grasp it. Removing sharp edges on the end of the instrument will reduce the chance of damaging the tissue. However if the object to be lifted is very small, the rounded edges may also prevent engagement with the object. It may be necessary therefore to have a 90° edge to pick up very small objects such as small diameter sutures (Figs. 3.4, 3.5, and 3.6).

T.H. Williamson, *Intraocular Surgery: A Basic Surgical Guide*,
DOI 10.1007/978-3-319-27990-9_3

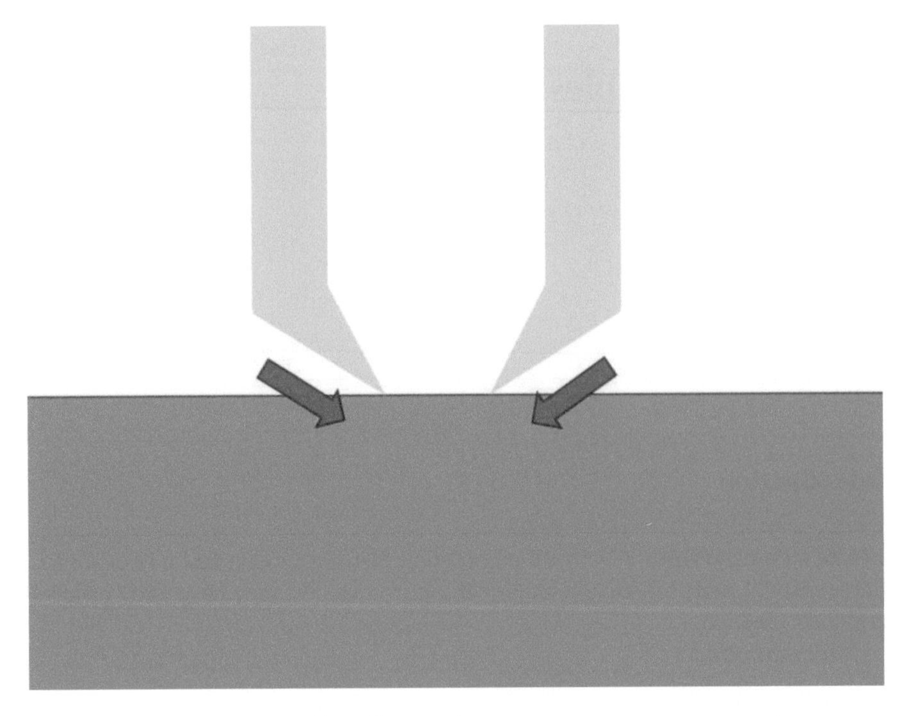

Fig. 3.1 Forceps are angled at 45° to allow the tips to penetrate a tissue on compression

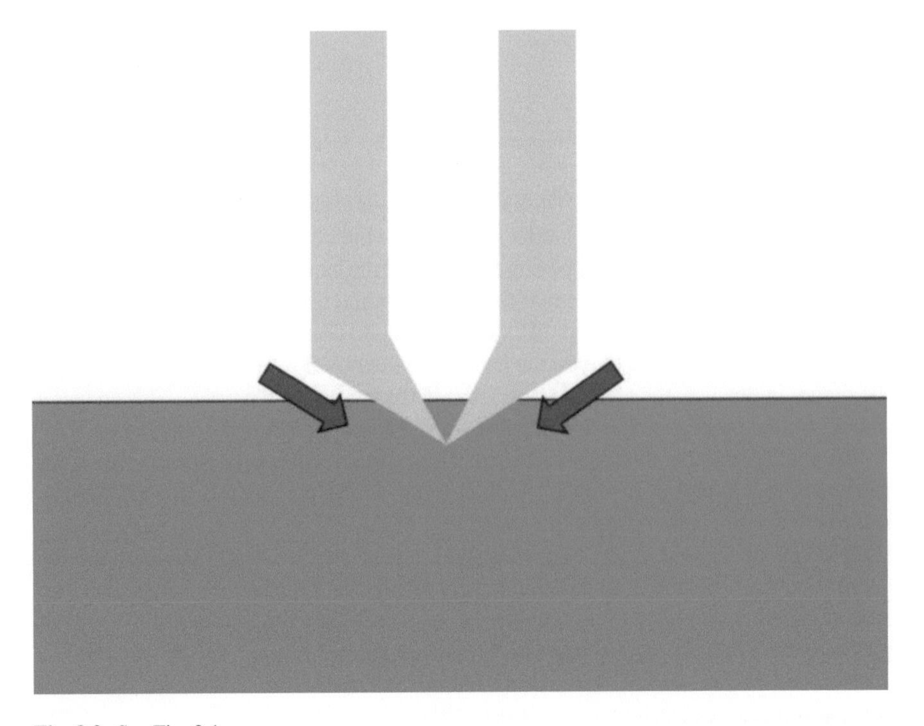

Fig. 3.2 See Fig. 3.1

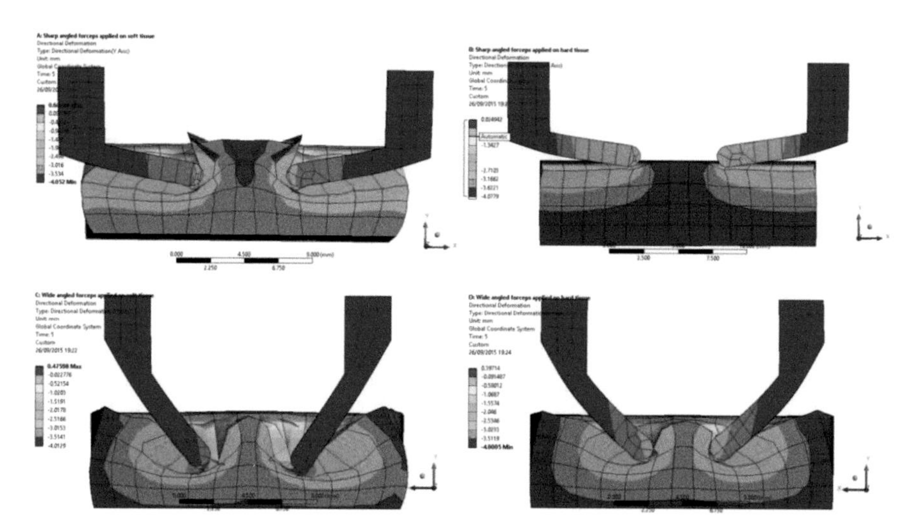

Fig. 3.3 FEA shows sharp and wide angled teeth displaced 4 mm downward into a soft tissue with Young's modulus of 100 Mpa and Poisson ratio of 0.49 and also into a hard tissue with Young's modulus of 1000 Mpa and Poisson ratio of 0.35. *Top left figure*: shows the effect of sharp angled teeth on a soft tissue, there is 83 % efficiency giving rise to 3.32 mm indentation. *Top right figure*: shows the effect of sharp angled teeth on a hard tissue, there is 43 % efficiency giving rise to 1. 73 mm indentation. *Bottom left figure*: shows the effect of wide angled teeth on a soft tissue, there is 98 % efficiency giving rise to 3.94 mm indentation. *Bottom right figure*: shows the effect of wide angled teeth on a hard tissue, there is 79 % efficiency giving rise to 3.16 mm indentation

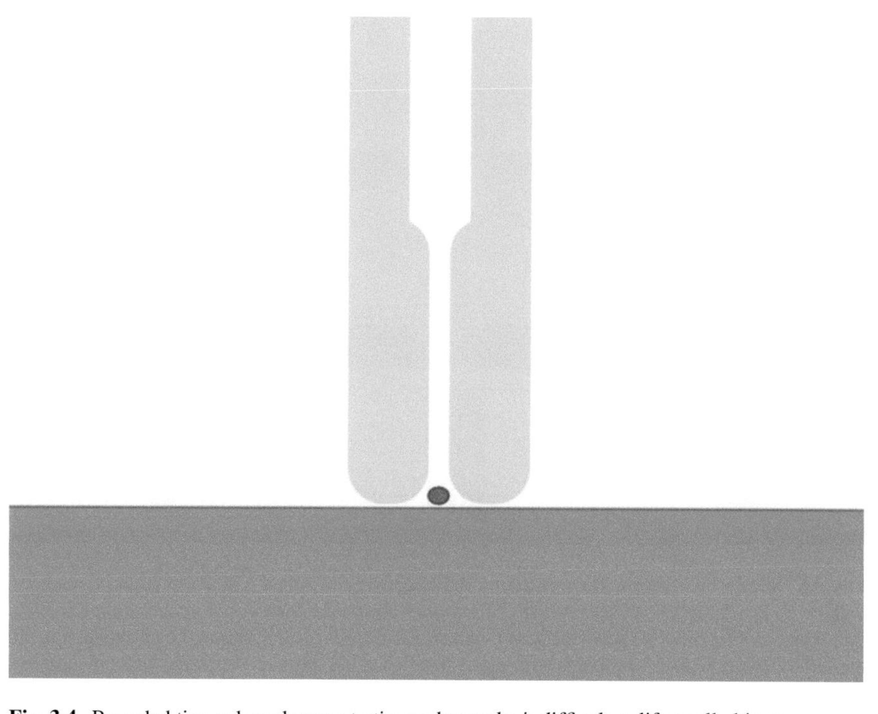

Fig. 3.4 Rounded tips reduce damage to tissues but make it difficult to lift small objects

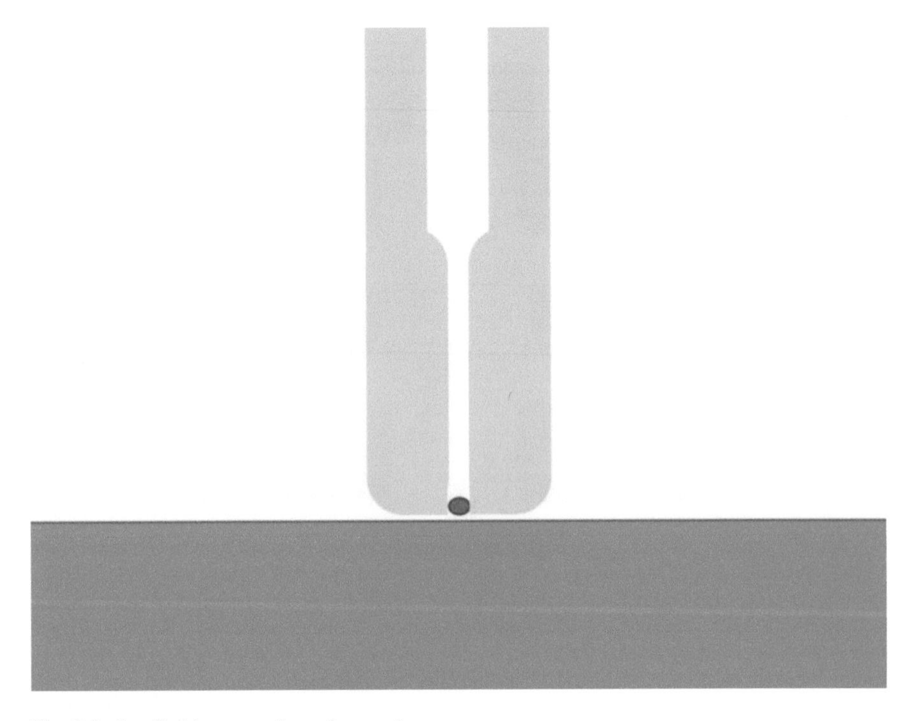

Fig. 3.5 Small objects require a sharper tip

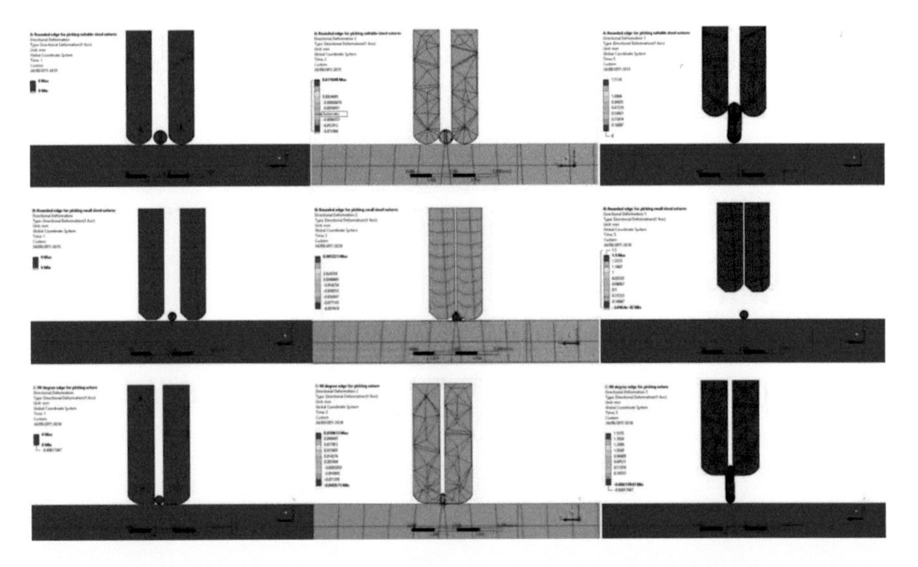

Fig. 3.6 Shows FEA results demonstrating the effectively of round and sharp edged forceps in picking up sutures of two different radii. *Left column* shows the forceps before attempting to pick the suture, *middle column* shows the grasping action and right column shows the pulling action on the suture. *Top row* shows a forceps with edges rounded at 0.8 mm radius is effective in picking up a suture that has a radius of 0.4 mm. *Middle row* shows a forceps with edges rounded at 0.8 mm radius fails to pick a smaller suture that has a radius of 0.25 mm. *Lower row* shows a 90^0 edge forceps is sufficiently effective in picking up a suture with a radius of 0.25 mm

For a simple forceps, applying more pressure to the handles increases the area of the contact of the tips, and increases the forces on the tissue. However the increased force required might damage the tissue or the object that the surgeon wishes to grasp, perhaps snapping a suture or tearing or crushing a tissue.

Often a platform is designed into the end of the forceps so that there is a broad area over which the object can be engaged. In the case of forceps with a platform the tissue or object can be confidently grasped with less force because a larger surface area is available. However, if excessive force is applied, this can induce flaring of the end of the forceps reducing its effectiveness. With some forceps a stop is introduced further up the shaft of the instrument to prevent such excessive pressure. This prevents excessive pressures distorting the platform only up to a certain point. If severely excessive pressure is applied the forceps will distort around this stop and separate the ends of the forceps once again.

It will be seen from this that an anxious surgeon who is heavy handed will reduce the effectiveness of the instrument in use, further adding to the poor surgeon's frustrations. Perhaps the surgeon will blame the instrument for their difficulties rather than their own surgical technique (Figs. 3.7, 3.8, 3.9, 3.10, 3.11, 3.12, and 3.13).

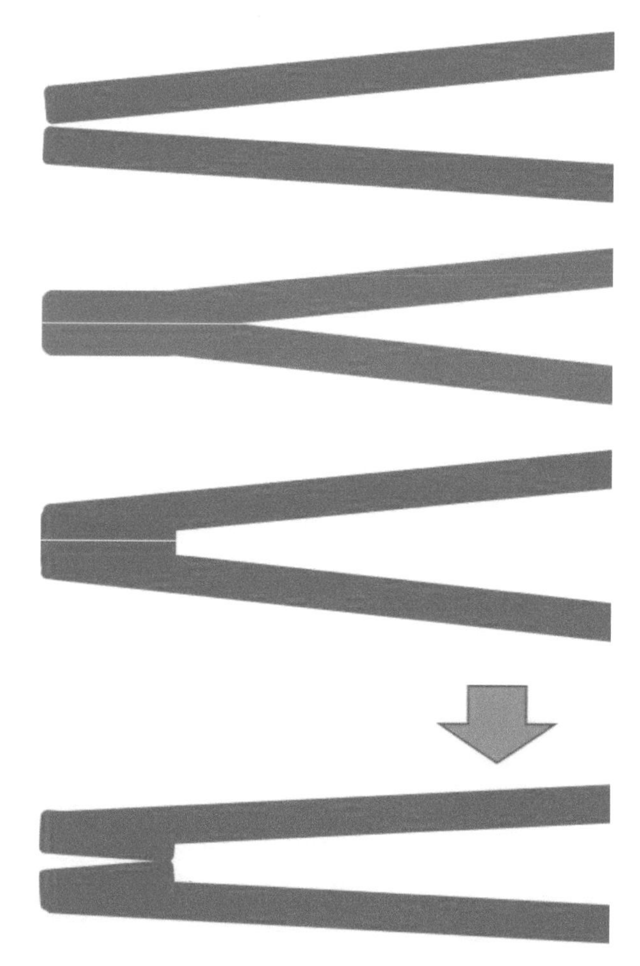

Fig. 3.7 Simple forceps have a very small area of contact

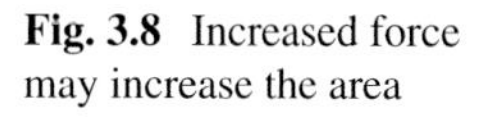

Fig. 3.8 Increased force may increase the area

Fig. 3.9 A plate can be used to increase the area

Fig. 3.10 Increased force can open up the forceps

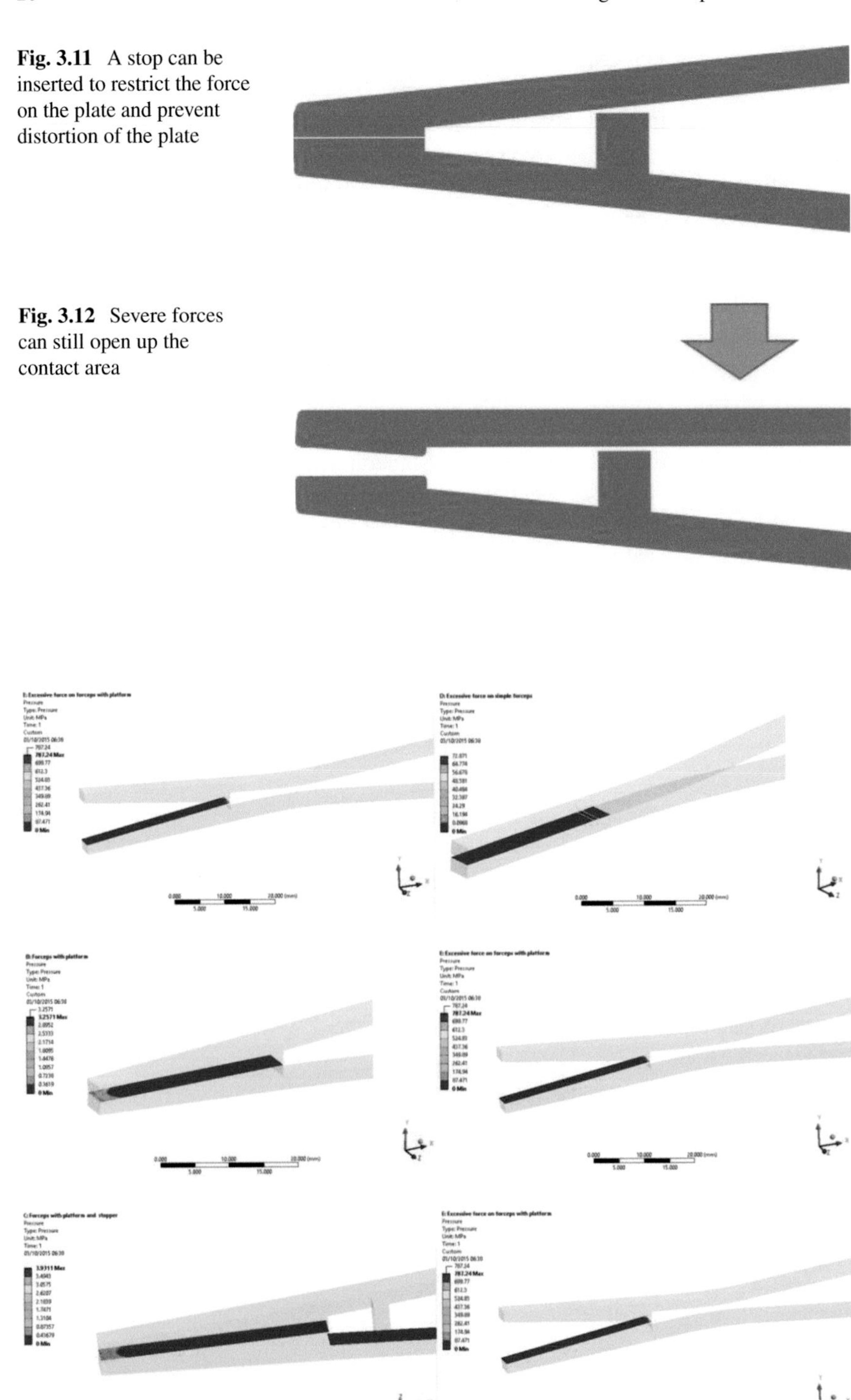

Fig. 3.11 A stop can be inserted to restrict the force on the plate and prevent distortion of the plate

Fig. 3.12 Severe forces can still open up the contact area

Visualisation

Often it is not possible with micro instruments to visualise the exact contact of the instrument with the tissue or object. There is nearly always a blind spot especially for many intraocular tasks and where the use of a microscope dictates the angle of view of the surgical field. The blind spot on a straight pair of forceps is often large, requiring the instrument tips to be made smaller to allow judgment of the contact with the tissue. The blind spot can be reduced by angulation of the tip to bring this into view. By curving the tips of the instrument, the blind spots are moved away from the point of contact, thereby improving visualisation (Figs. 3.14, 3.15, 3.16, and 3.17).

Mobile Tissue

Mobile and malleable tissues are better handled without the use of toothed forceps, because the teeth will create perforations, which can lead to tearing of the tissue. Instead the contact area of the forceps should have a serrated configuration. The soft tissue will deform into the undulations of the instrument, thereby allowing the tissue to be secured. In contrast a non-malleable tissue will not deform into the instrument leading to a small overall contact area and ineffective grasping of the tissue (Figs. 3.18, 3.19, 3.20, and 3.21).

Closure Mechanisms

There are different mechanisms to allow closure of the instrument tips for grasping or for cutting. The shafts may be apposed directly or indirectly through a hinging mechanism. For intra-ocular surgery wound sizes are kept to a minimum to maintain the stability of the globe, often restricting the use of instrumentation. Direct pressure systems are difficult to use inside the eye because they require a large range

Fig. 3.13 The figure shows FEA results demonstrating the magnitude and the distribution of contact pressures across the grasping surfaces of simple forceps, forceps with platforms and forceps with platforms and stoppers. *Top row*: shows 2 mm displacement of the handles of a closed simple forceps results in 8.51 MPa contact pressure at the tip of the forceps. Further displacement of the handles results in a shift of the contact pressure away from the tip of the forceps. *Middle row*: shows 2 mm displacement of the handles of a closed forceps with platform results in 3.25 MPa contact pressure at the tip of the forceps. Further displacement of the handles results in a shift of the contact pressure towards the posterior edge of the platform. *Bottom row*: 2 mm displacement of the handles of a closed forceps with platform and a stopper results in 3.93 MPa contact pressure at the tip of the forceps. Further displacement of the handles results in a shift of the contact pressure toward the stopper edge

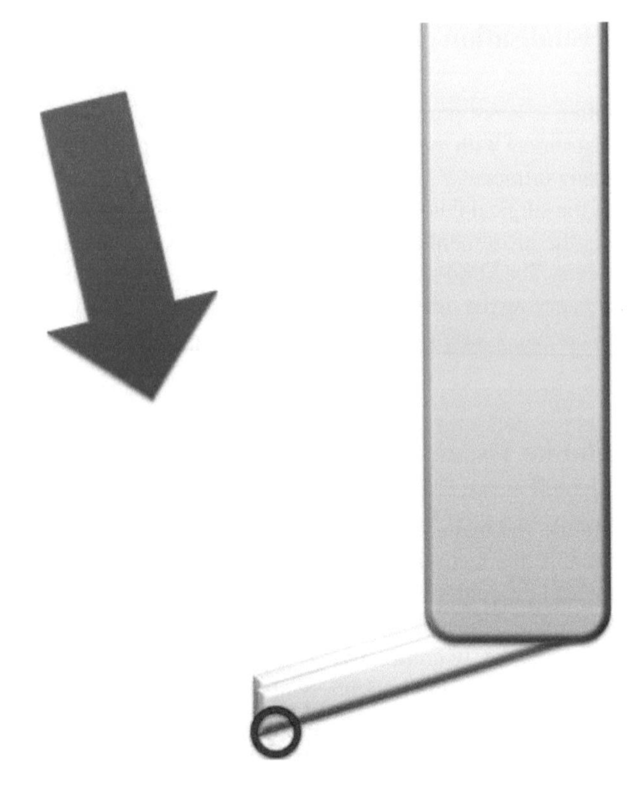

Fig. 3.14 The angle of viewing forceps may lead to blind spots

of movement for their action and therefore require a large wound size. They can only be advanced as far as the wound size will allow. A hinged system can be used through a small wound but has little range for advancement or a retraction of the instrument. Alternatively the instrument may employ a sleeve, which can be advanced from the action of a mechanism further up the shaft of the instrument. The sleeve's advancement will create approximation of the instrument tips. The sleeved system has the flexibility to be used through a small wound and permits a long range of insertion. The size of the instrument tip is however very small reducing its functionality, for example for the action of scissors. The forces that can be applied are also much reduced (Figs. 3.22, 3.23, and 3.24).

Angulation

Some instrument are restricted not only by the wound but by the spaces in which they are required to work. For example infusion and aspiration systems in cataract surgery have to work within the delicate capsule of the lens. The instruments need to be angulated to maximize their access. However that angulation may need to be changed depending on the area to be accessed. Angulation of instruments may

Fig. 3.15 The larger the instrument the larger the blind spot

Fig. 3.16 Curving the tips allows visualisation of the apposition of the tips

produce problems with the heel of the angle impacting on structures. It also means that the surgeon must change instruments to achieve a task. Another method is to create two wounds to allow access (see later) (Figs. 3.25, 3.26, 3.27, 3.28, 3.29, 3.30, 3.31, and 3.32).

Fig. 3.17 Keeping the instruments small improves the visualisation

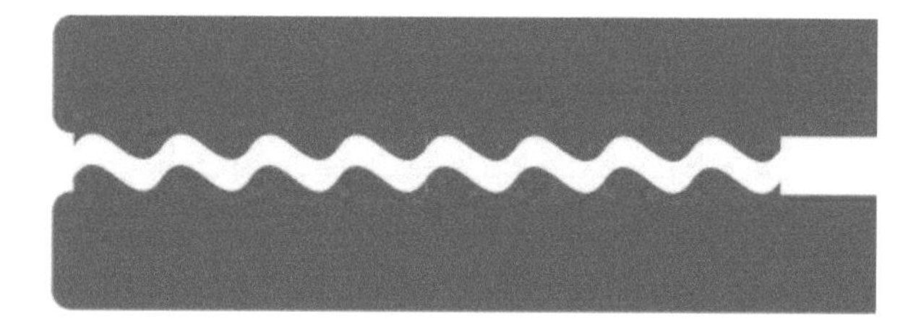

Fig. 3.18 Serrated forceps present a greater area for grasping tissue

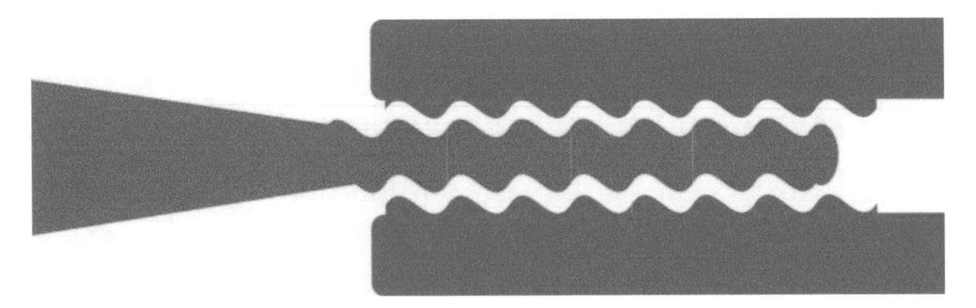

Fig. 3.19 Malleable tissues can distort into the serrations improving grip

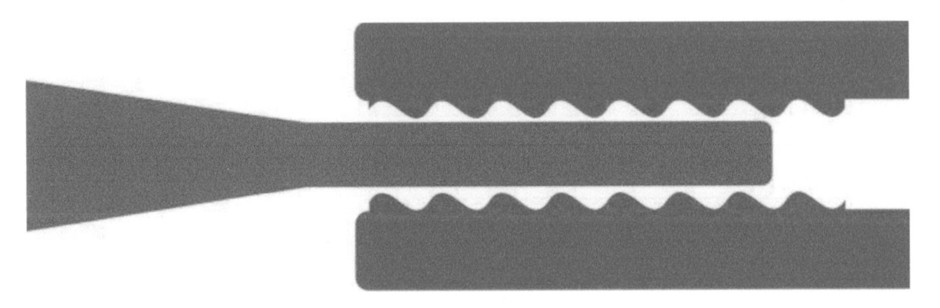

Fig. 3.20 Rigid tissues cannot distort causing a reduction in the area of contact with the tissue

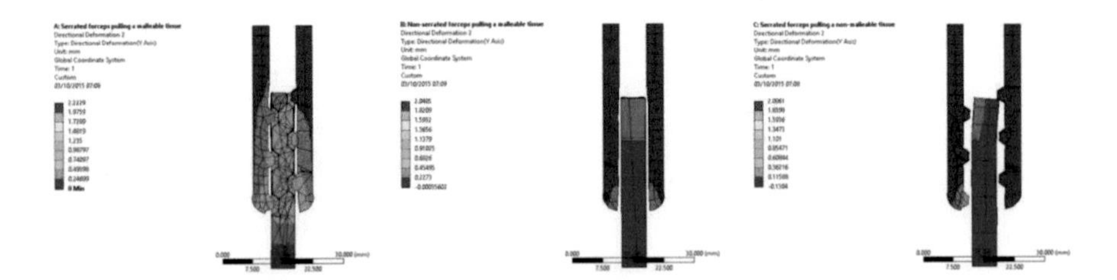

Fig. 3.21 Shows the results of FEA demonstrating the displacements attained with serrated forceps with and without undulation of the tissue and also the displacement achieved with non-serrated forceps. *Left*: shows a serrated forceps attaining 1.96 mm upward displacement in an undulated tissue when the forceps is displaced 2 mm upward (98 %) effectively. *Middle*: shows a non-serrated forceps attaining 0.45 mm upward displacement in the same tissue when the forceps is displaced 2 mm upward (22 %) effectively. *Right*: shows a serrated forceps attaining 0.30 mm upward displacement in an the same tissue but without achieving undulation when the forceps is displaced 2 mm upward (98 %) effectively

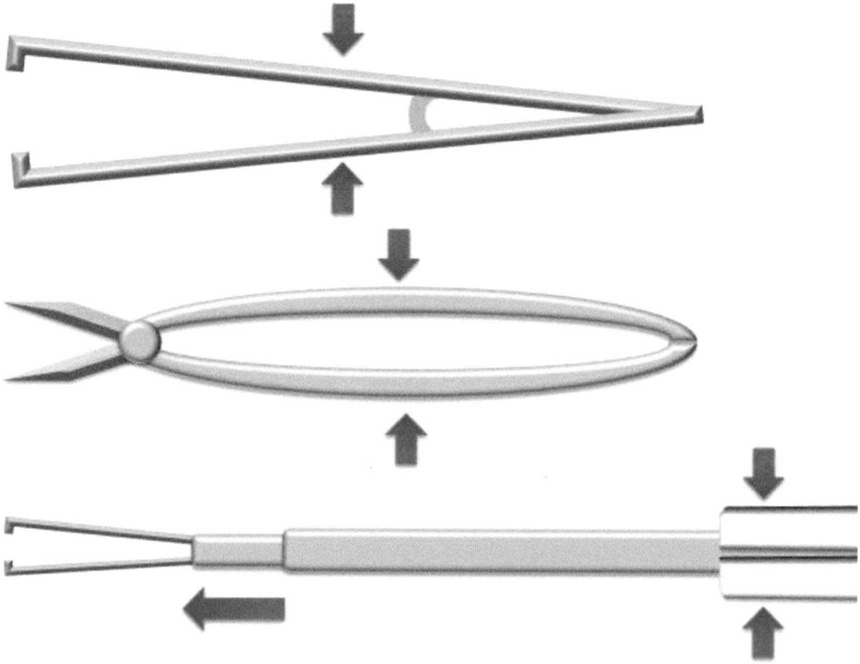

Fig. 3.22 Forceps can use different methods to appose the tips, direct compression of the shafts, compression via a hinge or compression from the effects of a moving sleeve

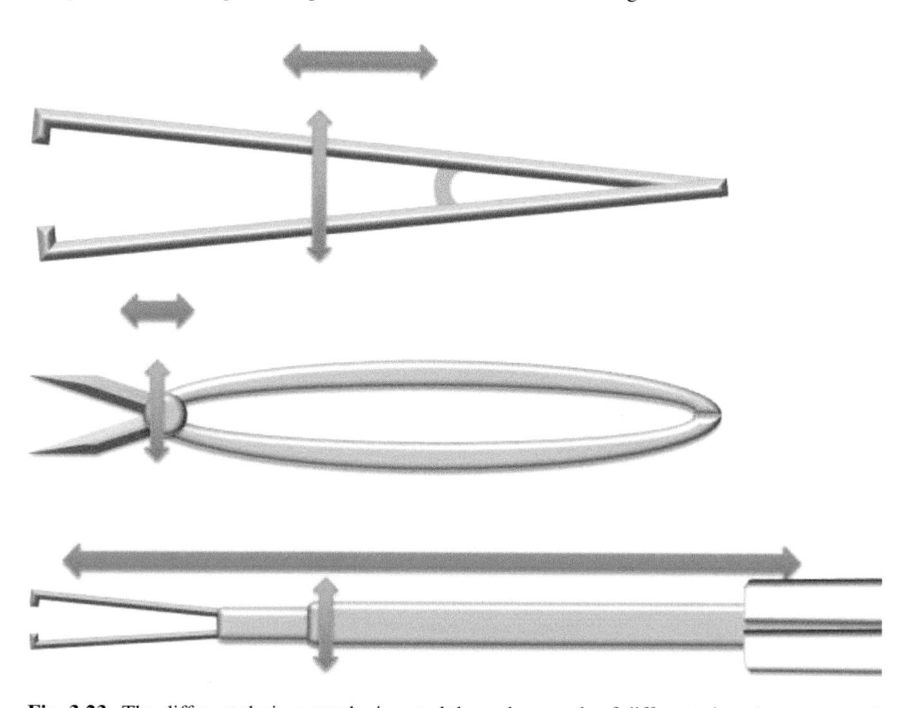

Fig. 3.23 The different designs can be inserted through wounds of different sizes (*green arrows*) but if the action of the instrument is to be maintained the ability to move the instrument in the wound is restricted depending upon the design

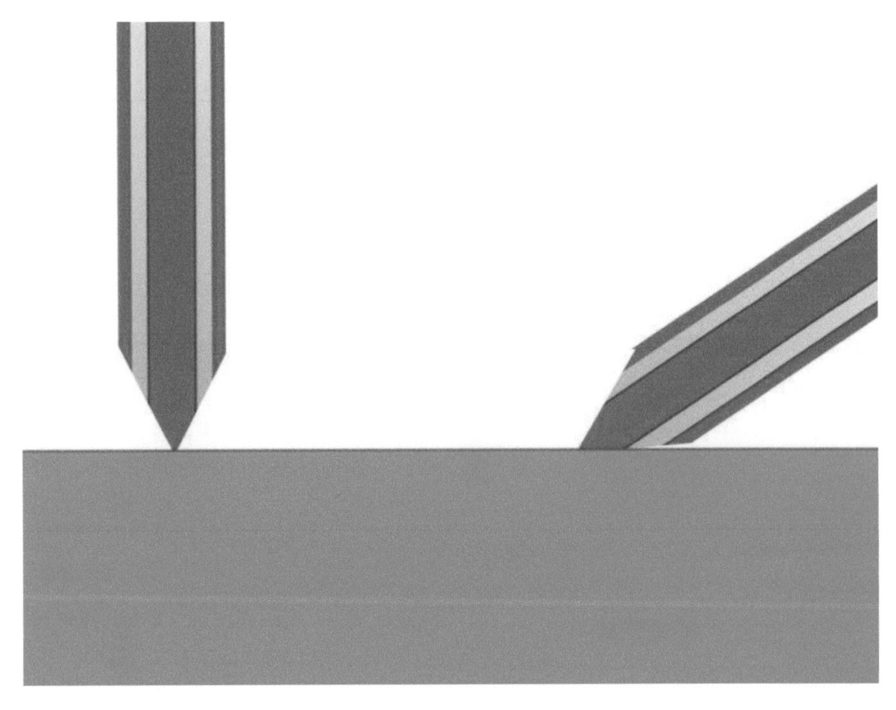

Fig. 3.24 Unipolar diathermy works by having both electrodes in the same tip, useful when inserting the instrument through small wounds. The instrument may work more effectively if angled as shown to allow the inner and outer electrode to be close to the tissue

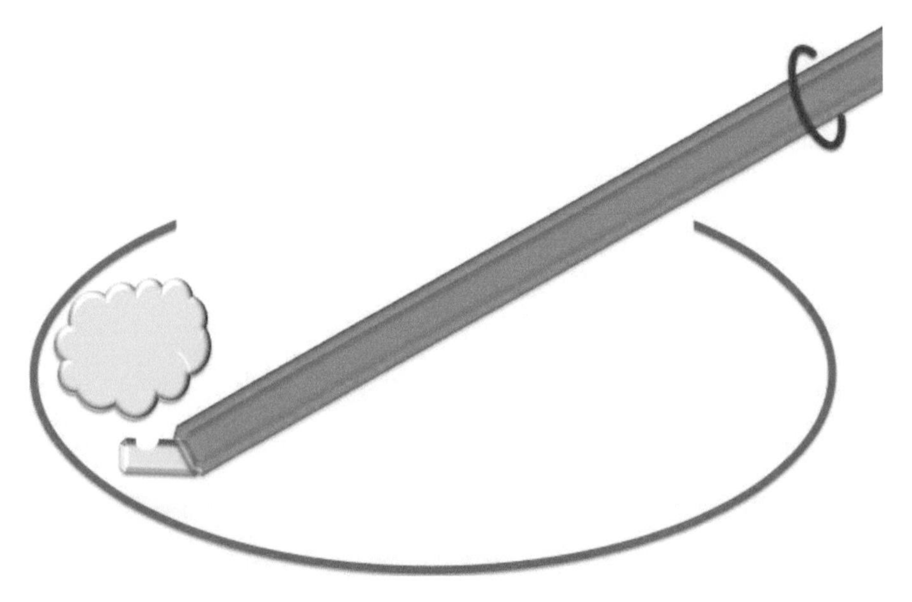

Fig. 3.25 The insertion of an instrument through a small would restricts the angle the surgeon can present the instrument within the tissue. Angulation of the instrument can be used to improve its function

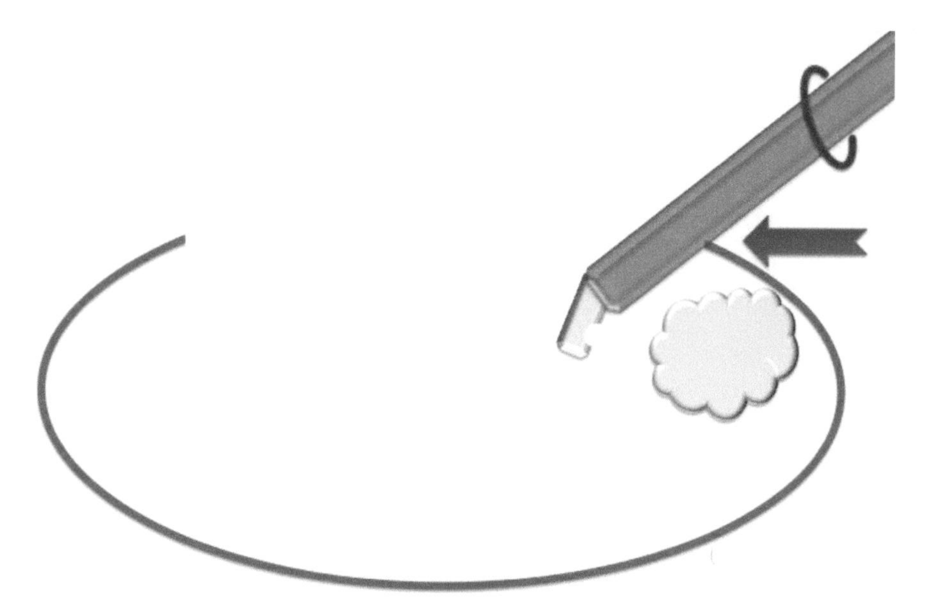

Fig. 3.26 The angulation for one area may not be appropriate for another site

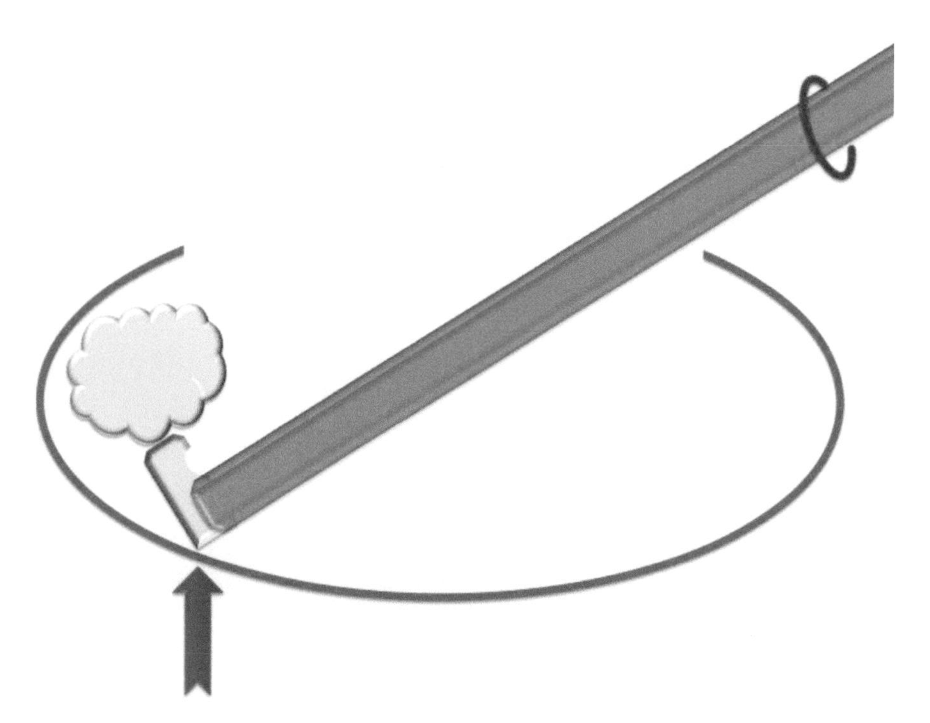

Fig. 3.27 Any angled instrument may cause tissue damage from the heel for the angle

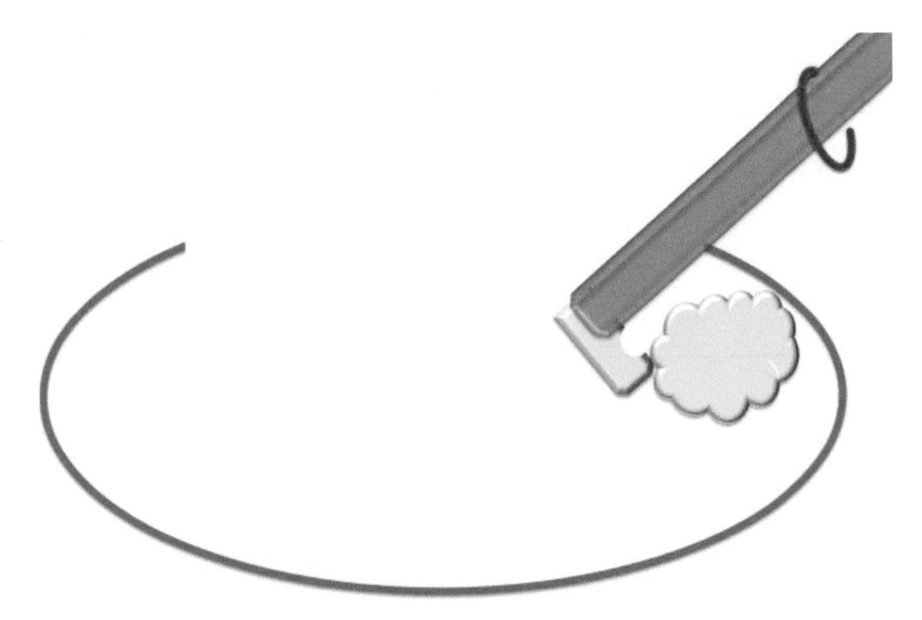

Fig. 3.28 The more acute angle helps when reaching tissues under the wound

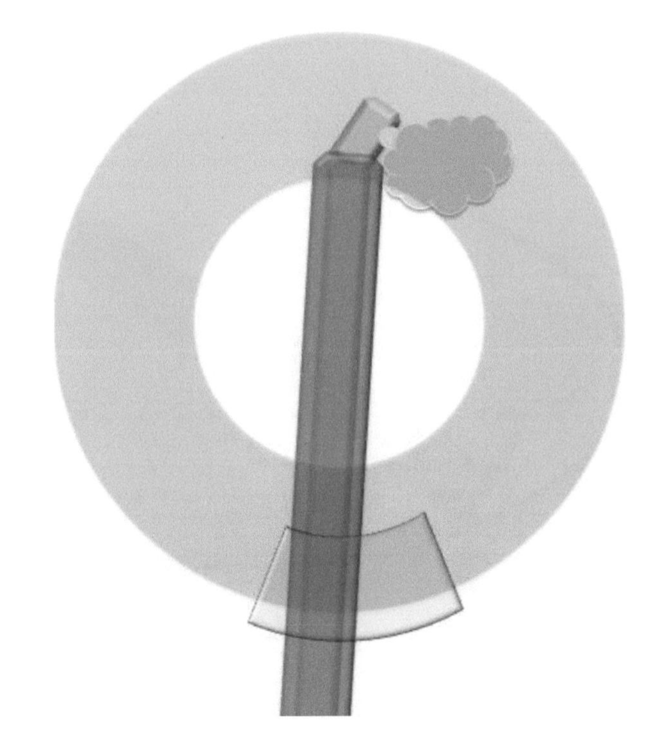

Fig. 3.29 Angulation is important on different planes horizontal and vertical

Fig. 3.30 Again the angulation has to be correct for the location

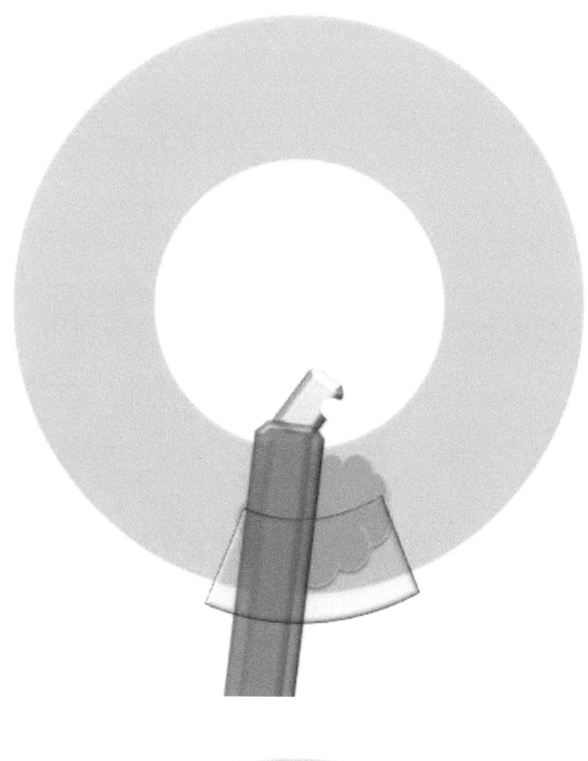

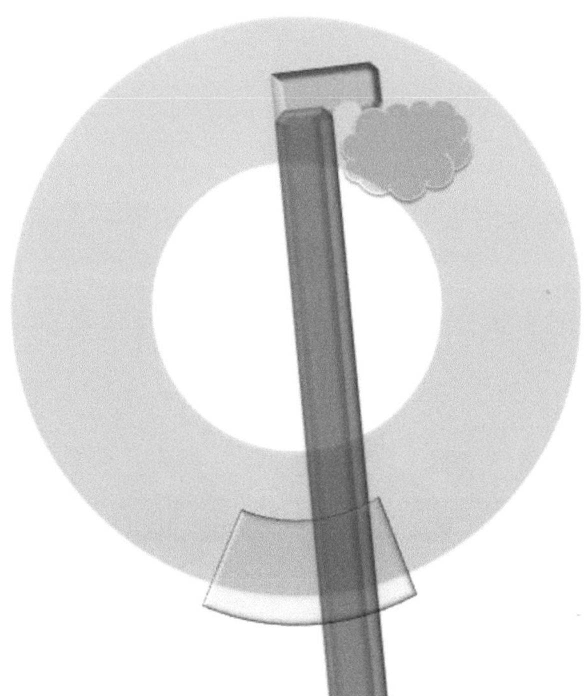

Fig. 3.31 Too acute angulation makes the instrument less effective in one site

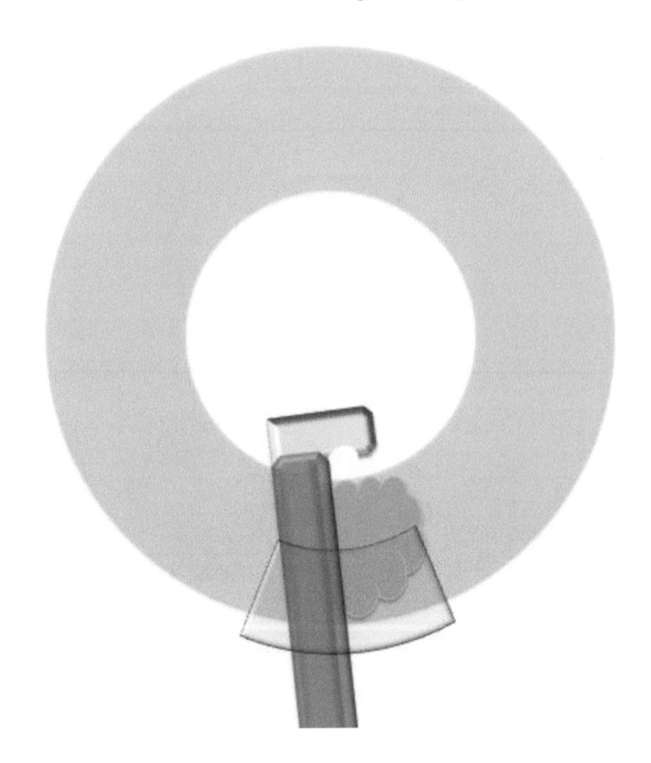

Fig. 3.32 The acute angle helps in the correct location

Chapter 4
Surgical Principles: Wounds and Tissue Manipulation

The surgeon should carefully consider certain principles when creating an incision. Wounds can be created in relatively stiff tissues or in relatively soft and malleable tissues: different principles may apply.

Incisions

A wound perpendicular to the surface of the tissue in any rigid structure is inherently unstable because pressure on any of the surfaces of the tissue will allow sliding of the wound causing an opening to appear. Most wounds in the eye are required to maintain the intraocular fluid contents, therefore any opening risks leakage of the intraocular fluids, causing a drop in intraocular pressure and risking complications. By sloping the wound, 2 of the surfaces become more stable, in addition a greater surface area is created within the wound producing more friction and prevent sliding. This configuration however is still open to instability from pressure on the 2 remaining surfaces. We will see later how use of a narrow wound can be used to make a sloped wound stable. A partially angled and vertical wound may also incur the same advantages and disadvantages. However, by using a partial vertical profile the length of the wound can be shortened whilst still obtaining the advantage of some stability (Figs. 4.1, 4.2, and 4.3).

A Chevron wound, sloping in two different directions is inherently stable, because pressure on all 4 surfaces cannot open the wound. In addition the cross-sectional area of the wound is again increased whilst keeping the overall area of tissue disruption to a minimum. A disadvantage is that these wounds are difficult to suture satisfactorily should some instability be found (Fig. 4.4).

When dealing with the eye most of the surfaces are not flat but are curved. Despite this, essentially the same principles apply with instability of wounds

T.H. Williamson, *Intraocular Surgery: A Basic Surgical Guide*,
DOI 10.1007/978-3-319-27990-9_4

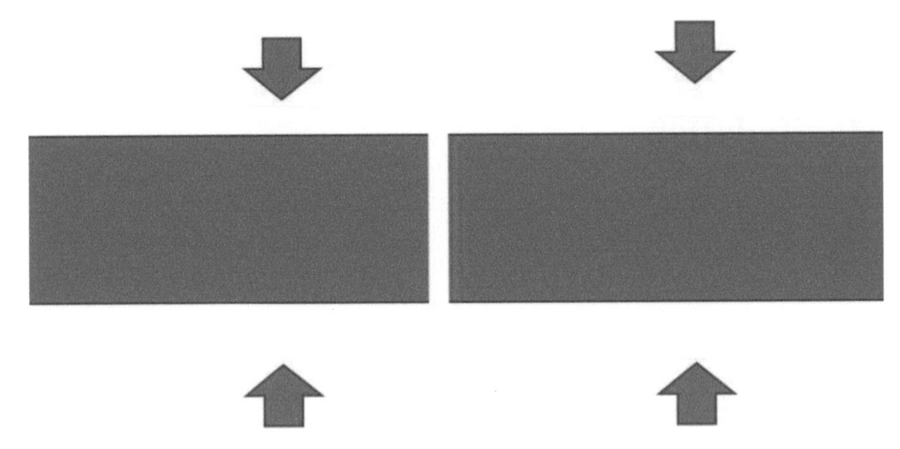

Fig. 4.1 A vertical perpendicular wound is unstable because pressure on 4 locations (*arrows*) can cause movement and because the area of the wound surface (for friction in the wound) is at the minimum

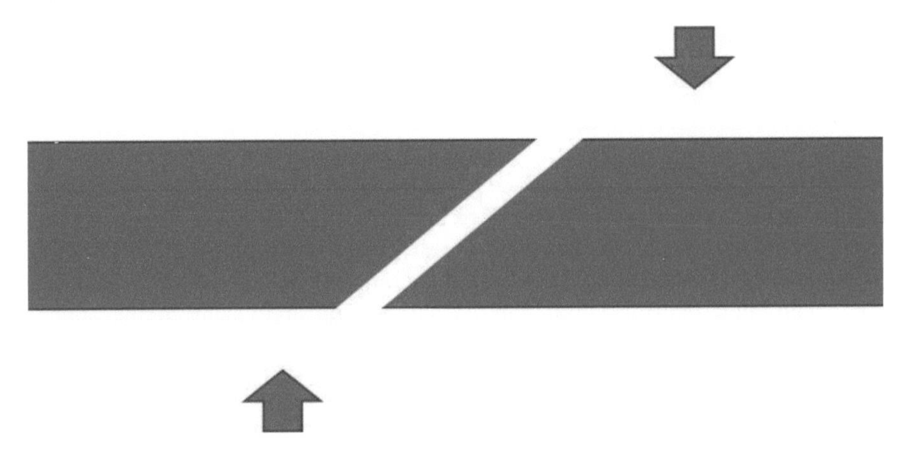

Fig. 4.2 A diagonal wound is only destabilsed by pressure on two locations and increases the surface area of the wound

perpendicular to the curve and increased stability when the wounds are shelved into the curve (Figs. 4.5 and 4.6).

Wounds however do not exist only in 2 dimensions, and the 3-D profile of the wound also affects its stability. A simple shelved wound is often used in anterior segment surgery. This will not usually require suturing. Note that an incision, which you believe is straight, may in fact be curved because of the way the tissue moves ahead of the blade in the tissue, following the spherical shape of the structures of the eye.

There are two orifices, which must open, internal and external. A tangential line can be drawn from the fixed ends of the wound at the external orifice when looking at the wound *en face*, if this line does not cross the internal orifice, it is very difficult for the internal and external orifices to open simultaneously without an external

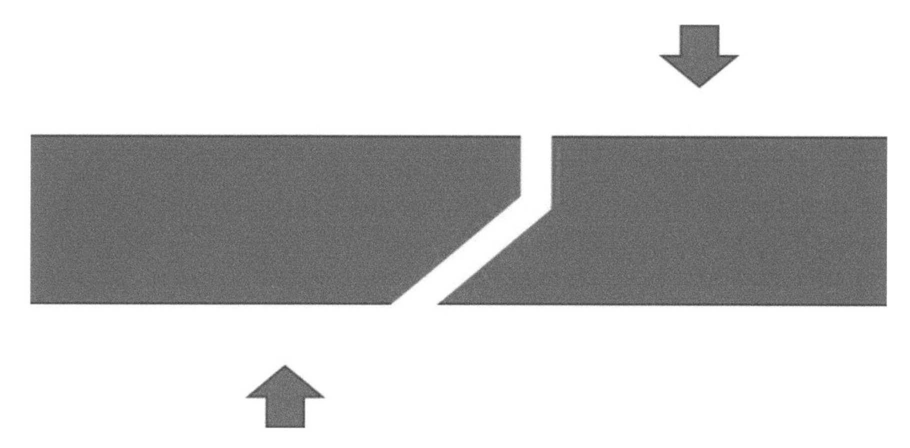

Fig. 4.3 A partially sloped wound can achieve some of the advantages of sloped wound and may be easier to suture

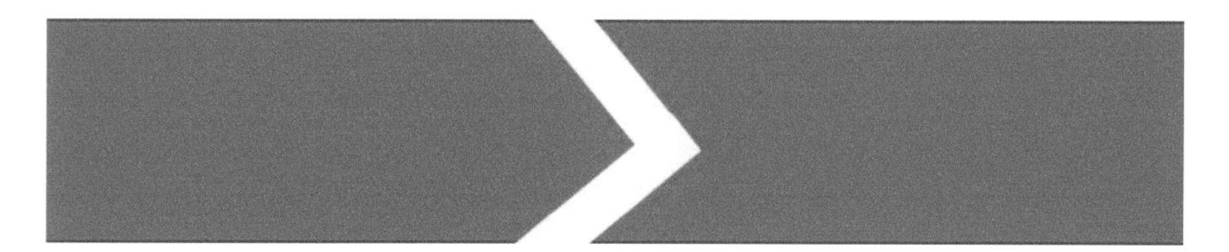

Fig. 4.4 A chevron shaped wound is stable in all directions

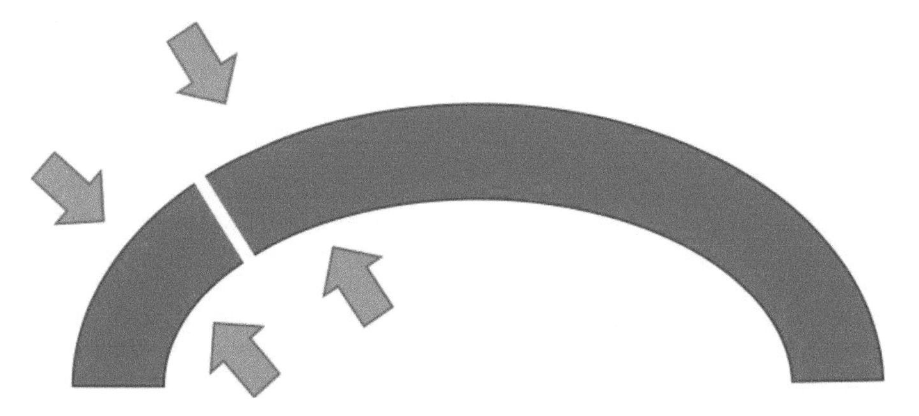

Fig. 4.5 The perpendicular wound is unstabe in a curved tissue

force (e.g., the surgeon actively opening the wound). Therefore a narrow, long shelved wound in a spherical object is very stable, explaining why anterior segment wounds can be left unsutured in cataract surgery. If the wound is made too wide and not long enough, the tangential line from the fixed points of the external curve will cross the internal curve and it is very easy for the wound to separate opening the

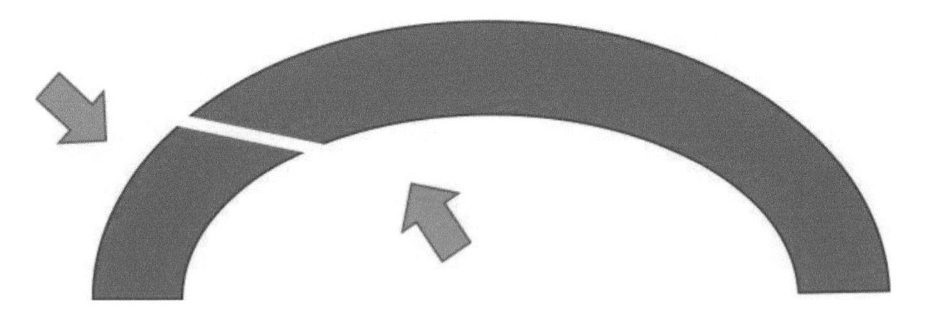

Fig. 4.6 The sloped wound is more stable

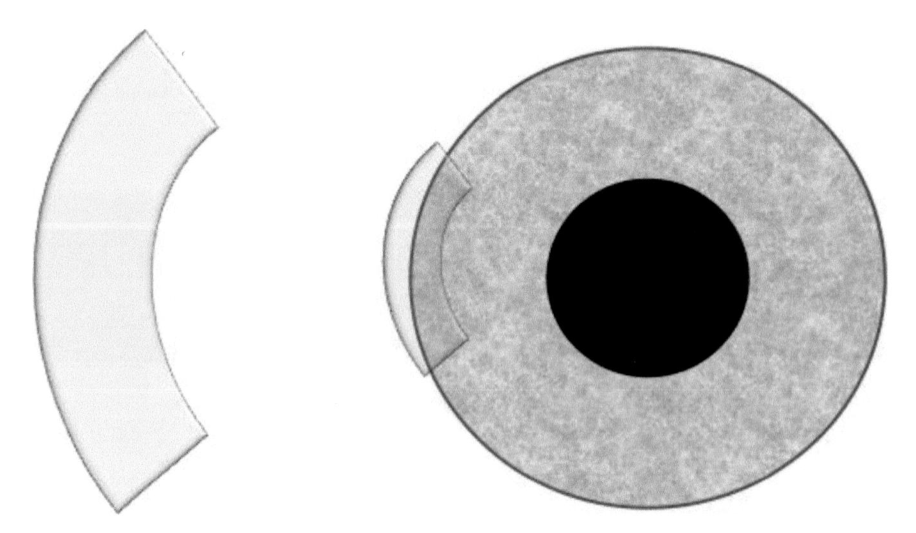

Fig. 4.7 Wounds in the eye are also influenced by their width and length

internal orifice and leaking intraocular fluids. We will see later how a simple suturing technique will reposition the tangential line and re-stabilise the wound (Figs. 4.7 and 4.8).

Incisions are made by the action of instrumentation. The design of such instrumentation influences the wound that is created. A narrow blade with equal length along its angulated sides will create a thin slice directly through a tissue. There will be minimal tissue compression and displacement by the blade. However the narrow angulation reduces the stability of the blade as it passes through the tissue increasing the chance of deviation off the line of the incision.

When the angulation of the blade sides become less acute and the blade becomes broader, more tissue displacement will occur and a broader wound will be created. The blade will be more stable however as it incises the tissue. The increase in the angle will increase the friction on the advancement of the blade and increase the

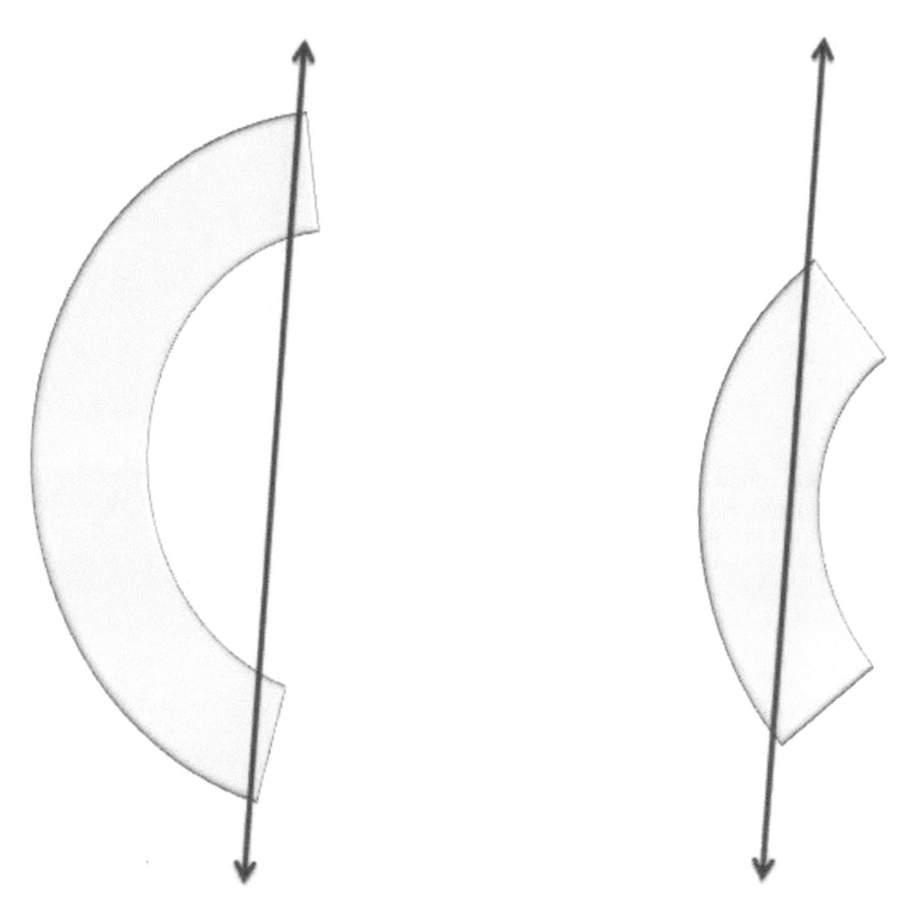

Fig. 4.8 A wound needs to rotate along a line from the corners of its outer incision to open. If the line crosses within the arc of the inner incision (*left*) the wound will leak. If the line does not cross within the inner arc the tissues are still apposed and the wound will not leak

force required to create the wound. An asymmetric profile to the blade, for example one side is angulated and the other not, will create forces on the blade, which will deviate it from the straight path. The tangential force on the angled side will direct the blade away from this side. This causes a curved wound, unless forces are applied to the blade to prevent this (Figs. 4.9, 4.10, 4.11, 4.12, 4.13, and 4.14).

A triangular blade applies forces laterally in addition to the forces for advancement of the blade through the tissue. The greater the width of the blade the greater is the force being exerted laterally and the more difficult the blade is to insert into the tissue (Figs. 4.15 and 4.16).

Not all tissues are rigid however, and incisions will vary in malleable or mobile tissue. Consideration must be made to the effects of a blade on a mobile tissue which is fixed along one border. Because the tissue is able to move during the action

Fig. 4.9 The profile of a blade effects how it will interact with a tissue

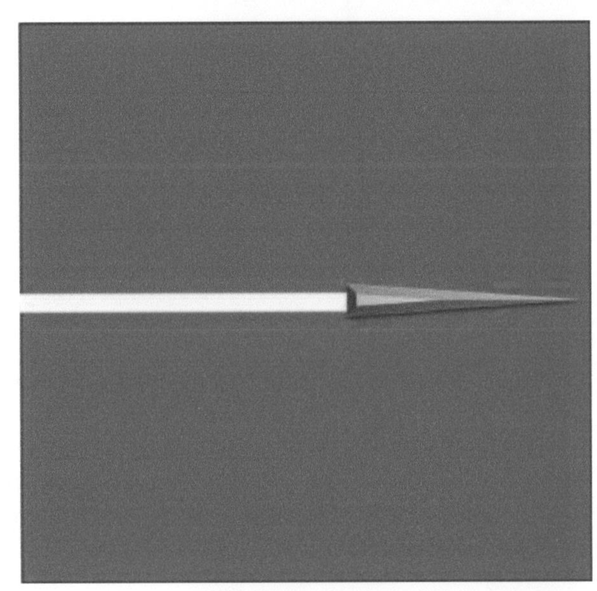

Fig. 4.10 A narrow blade with equal sides will pass through tissue in a straight line, displacing the tissue only slightly. Resistance will be low

Fig. 4.11 A broad blade has different characteristics

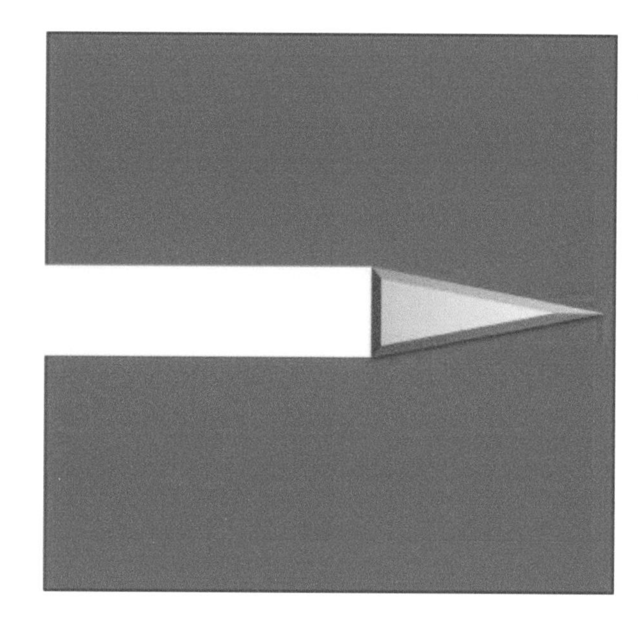

Fig. 4.12 The blade displaces more tissue and suffers more resistance but is less prone to alterations in its course and may give a more reliably straight course

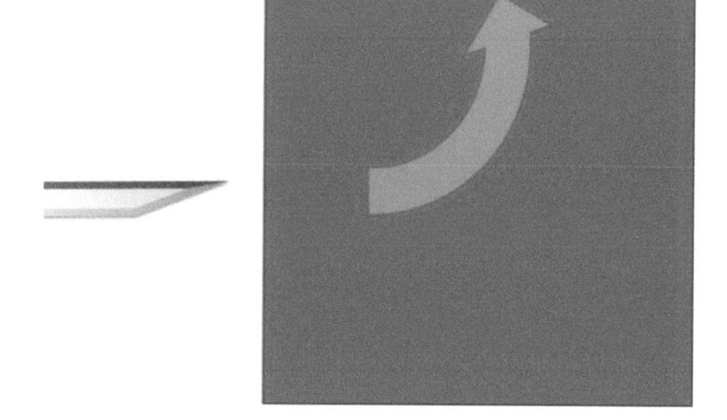

Fig. 4.13 If the blade is asymmetric with one side angled more compared to the other the vector of action of the blade causes the blade to take a curved path away from the angled side

of the blade, the tissue tends to move towards the fixed border. In effect the wound is curved away from the fixed edge. This is seen for example when trying to cut conjunctiva from the edge of the corneal limbus. The conjunctiva is fixed at the limbus and is free to move in the fornixes. Using scissors to cut the conjunctiva, the wound will be naturally drawn towards the fornixes. The surgeon will have to apply a force to counter this natural movement in order to keep the wound at the edge of the limbus (Figs. 4.17, 4.18, and 4.19).

Fig. 4.14 The wound becomes curved

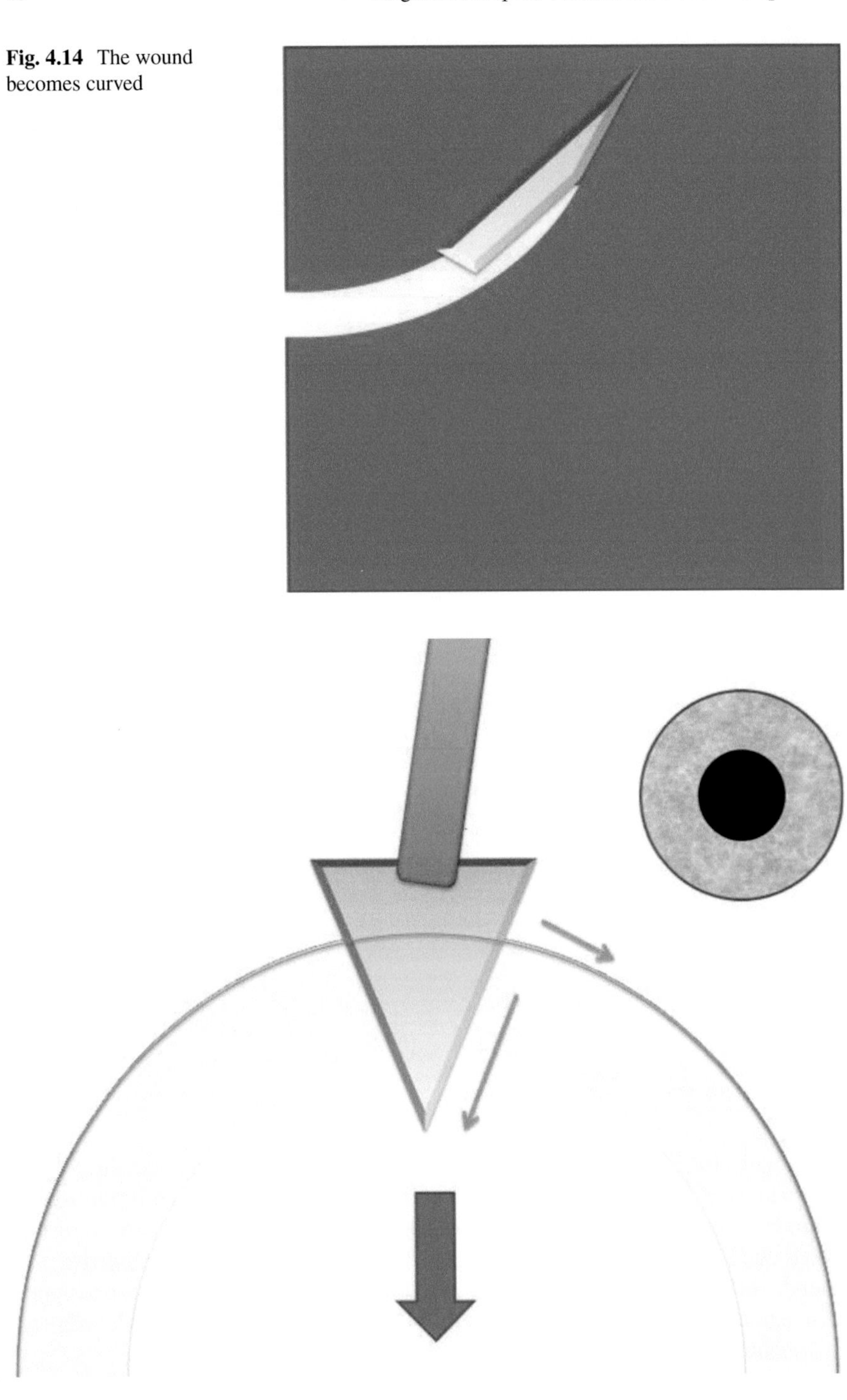

Fig. 4.15 The profile of a blade affects its action with a triangular blade distributing force laterally in addition

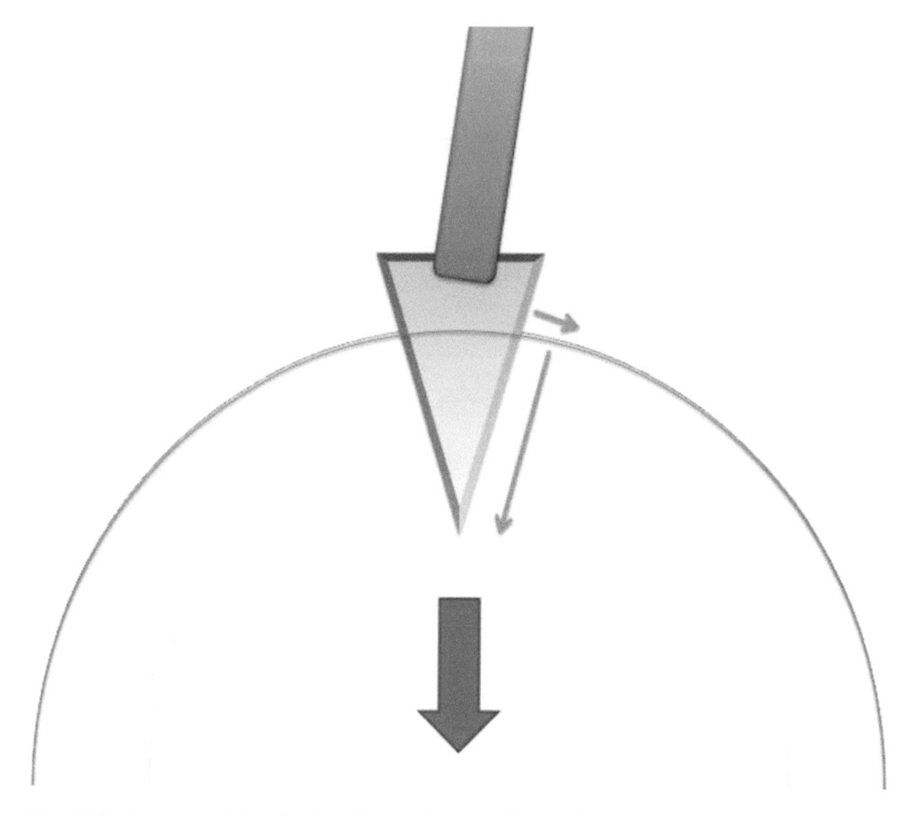

Fig. 4.16 A narrower blade has less force going laterally and is easier to insert

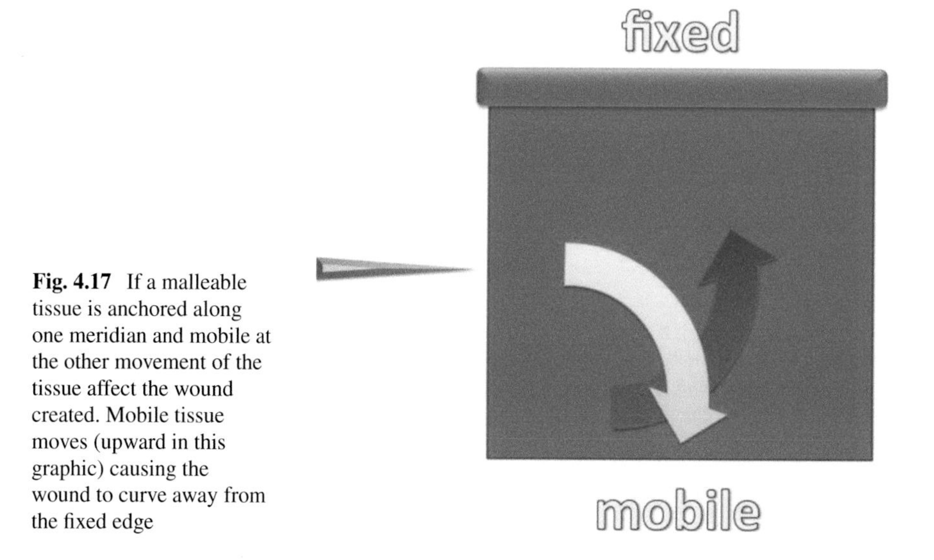

Fig. 4.17 If a malleable tissue is anchored along one meridian and mobile at the other movement of the tissue affect the wound created. Mobile tissue moves (upward in this graphic) causing the wound to curve away from the fixed edge

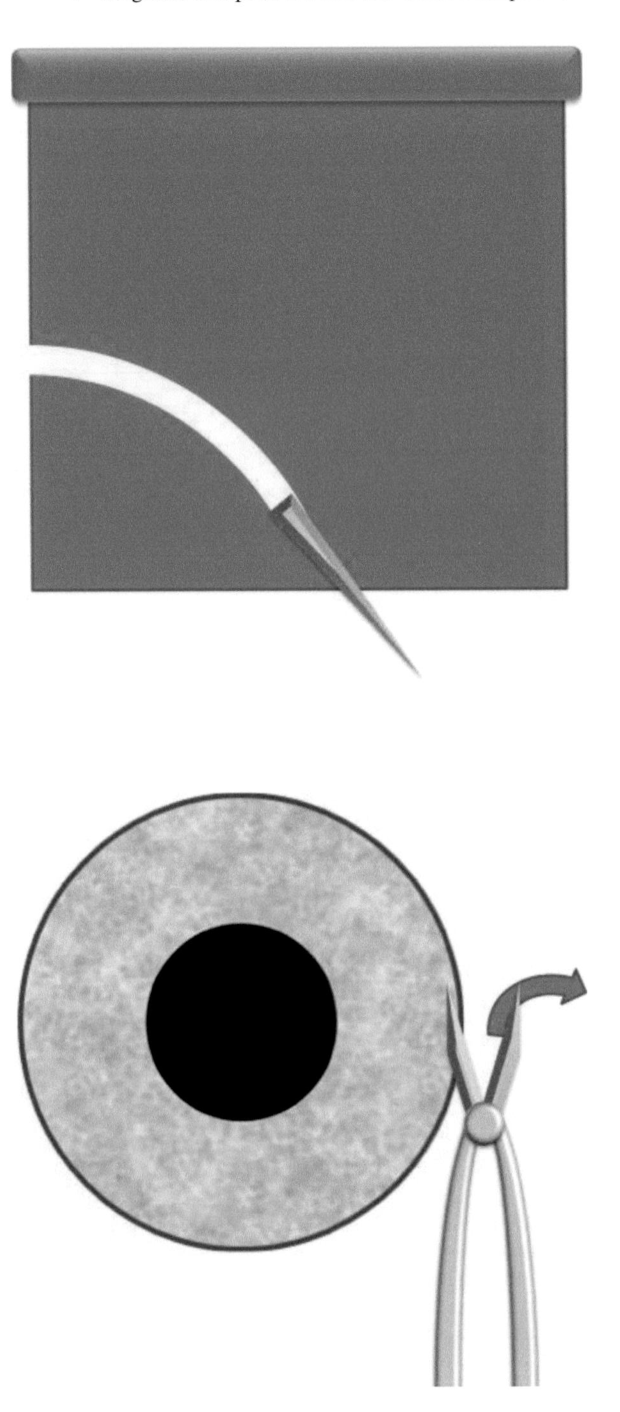

Fig. 4.18 A curved wound is created even with a symmetrical blade

Fig. 4.19 Cutting the conjunctiva where the tissue is anchored at the limbus and mobile in the fornices cause the incision to be drawn away from the limbus requiring counter pressure on the instrument by the surgeon

FEA, Appreciation of the Surgical Planes in Microsurgery

Microscopes are used to enhance tissue visualisation and to identify precise anatomic details. However, stereo-acuity and depth of perception are reduced with increasing magnification, as a result small degrees of tilts in the surgical plane may not be appreciated by the ophthalmic surgeon. Failure to align microsurgical tools in the plane parallel to the iris while initiating and continuing certain surgical manoeuvres may lead to suboptimal outcomes. Therefore it is essential for the surgeon to ensure that the eyeball is in a neutral position so that the iris plane is parallel to the floor. If keeping the eyeball in the neutral position is not possible, because of the effect of local or general anaesthetics, then the surgeon will need to adjust his or her manoeuvres to match the tilt in the iris plane by bringing the eyeball to the neutral position using assisting forceps or by using his tools in a way that matches the plane of the iris. The following are examples of microsurgical procedures that need to be carried out at a plane that is parallel to the iris.

Corneal Section and the Surgical Plane

Clear corneal sections should be performed with the keratome held parallel to the iris plane. If the keratome is held inadvertently at an angle to the iris plane the internal and the external orifices of the section will not be aligned with the limbus, with one side of the wound being very close to the limbus and the other side too advanced into the clear corneal zone. Variability in incision length may pose surgical challenges for the rest of the surgery, such as decreased instrument mobility, decreased visibility due to corneal striae and hydration, postoperative leak, increased astigmatism and even increased risk of endophthalmitis (Fig. 4.20).

Rigid and Malleable

In the circumstances where rigid tissues are opposed to elastic tissues, the 2 tissues may react differently to the instrumentation. A blade inserted into a rigid tissue will cut this tissue but may push elastic and mobile tissue away from the blade tip without penetrating it. This feature is classically used in neurosurgery to create a burr hole in the skull. The burr oscillates rather than rotating only in one direction. This means that the burr can drill into the rigid bone of the skull, but should it encounter the elastic dura mater, the dura will be able to move with the blade back and forward without being penetrated or torn. In the eye the same phenomenon is seen when inserting a blade through the sclera, and into the choroid. The choroid is elastic and will move away from the blade so that a large wound is found in the sclera but only a small penetration is found in the choroid (Figs. 4.21 and 4.22).

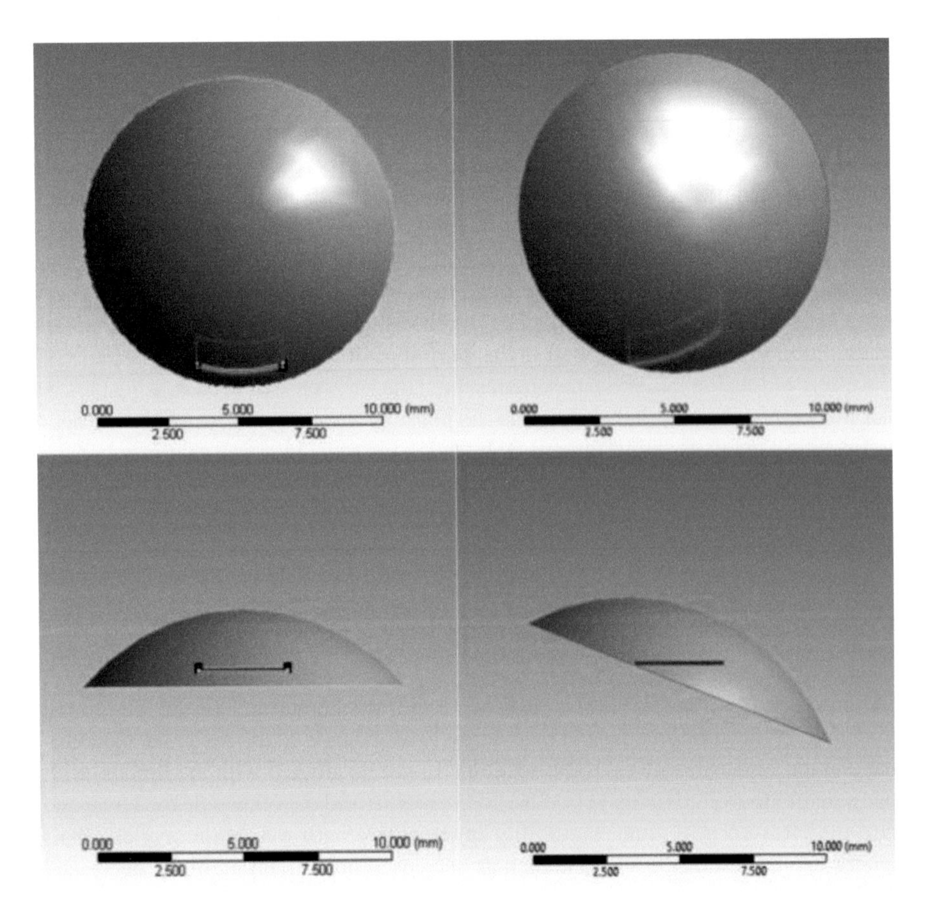

Fig. 4.20 FEA *Left image* shows a clear corneal section performed with the keratome held parallel to the iris plane; *right image* shows a clear corneal section performed with a keratome held parallel to the floor in an eye that has a 20° tilt to the right, resulting in an asymmetrical corneal section. *Top row* is the top view of the cornea as it appears under the microscope and the *bottom row* is the side view of the cornea

Scissors

Scissors function by passing 2 asymmetric blades across each other. The asymmetry of the blades would under natural forces allow the blades to separate preventing them opposing and cutting the tissue. To avoid this the hinge is designed to apply a strong counter force keeping the blades together. These opposing forces have the effect of distorting the tissue during the incision. In a rigid tissue and this will eventually create an S-shaped profile to the wound. This shape will create some stability, but in its creation the tissues are crushed and distorted in comparison to the wound created by a single sharp blade. Therefore scissors are now rarely used in tissues whose structural integrity is crucial for example the cornea (Fig. 4.23).

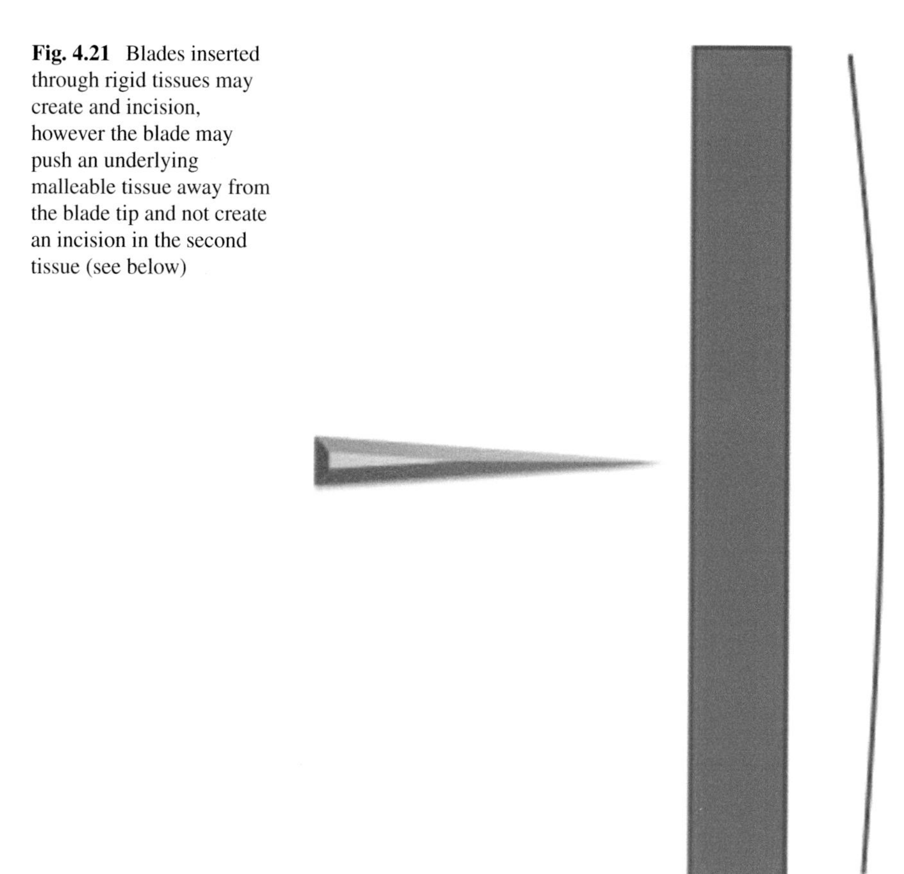

Fig. 4.21 Blades inserted through rigid tissues may create and incision, however the blade may push an underlying malleable tissue away from the blade tip and not create an incision in the second tissue (see below)

Loose tissues such as conjunctiva are easily distorted risking irregularity in the wound profile. For example care must be taken when lifting such a tissue to cut it. If grasping the tissue pinch the tissue in a parallel fashion to the direction of the cut. Any compression of the tissue will then be parallel to the wound maintaining a straight wound. In contrast if you pinch the tissue perpendicular to the wound the tissue in the centre of the wound will be pulled towards the grasping instrument, creating a curved wound (Figs. 4.24, 4.25, and 4.26).

Lamellar Wounds

Lamellar tissues have characteristics, which the surgeon can exploit. An incision perpendicular to the lamellae passes through the tissue in a straight line. However an oblique incision is deflected slightly every time the blade transits from a softer lamella to a harder lamella, eventually this encourages the blade to take a curved path and end up passing parallel to the lamellae. This can be used to help make a needle pass along a thin lamellar tissue e.g., sclera, without penetrating the sclera

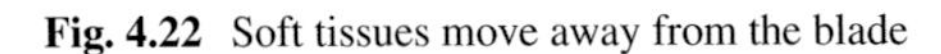

Fig. 4.22 Soft tissues move away from the blade

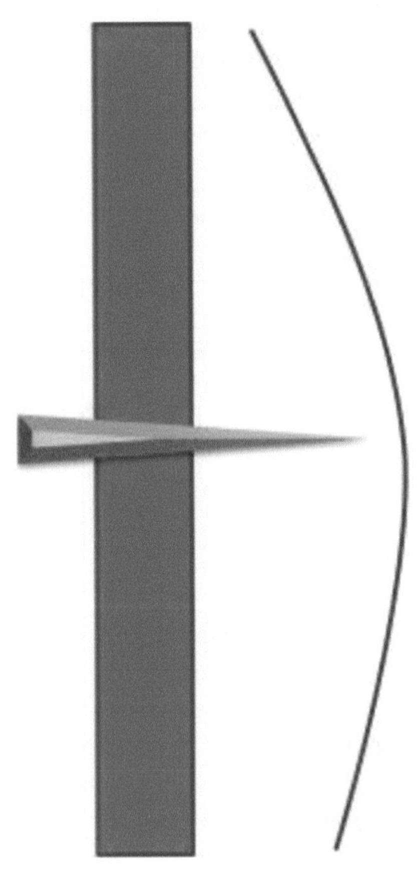

(for example for suturing into the sclera). The lamellae also guide dissection of the tissue when creating a flap, e.g., in trabeculectomy (Figs. 4.27 and 4.28).

Curved Wounds

The curved nature of the globe needs to be considered when forces are applied to an incision. When a curved wound is elevated the tissue hinges along a line between the ends of the wound, this creates a downward force along this line which will flatten the curve. In addition, the ends of the wound are forced apart. If the wound has a perpendicular depth, the forces of elevation on the external wound twist the ends of the wounds. The wound has a force which tries to make it flat along a line passing from the internal edge of the wound. The elevation therefore of a curved flap causes considerable distortion to the globe (Figs. 4.29, 4.30, 4.31, and 4.32).

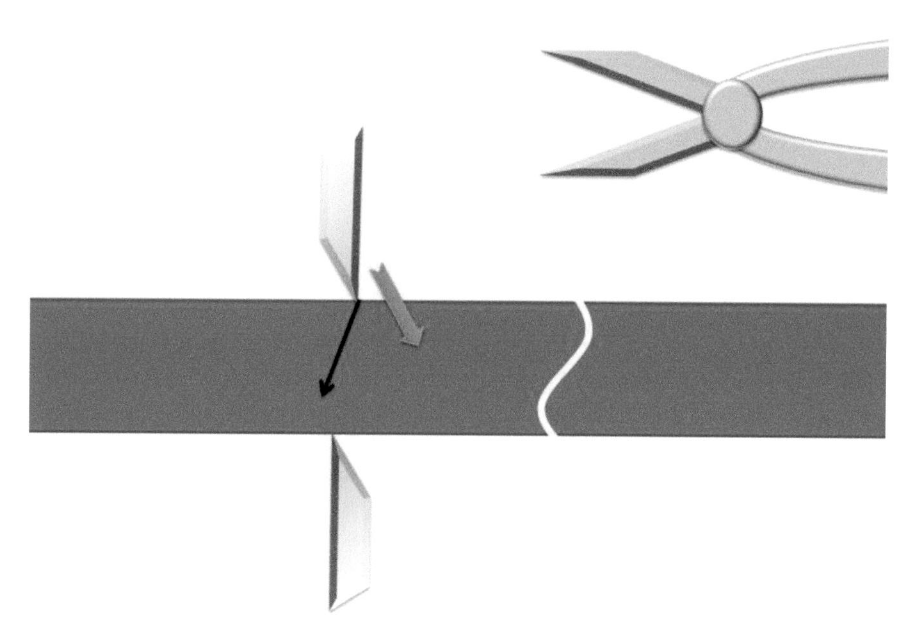

Fig. 4.23 Scissors work by forcing two opposing blades to pass close to each other. Vectors of the action of the blades is to direct the blades away from each other. A force is applied to the blades to counteract this. The conflict of forces and vectors creates an S shaped wound

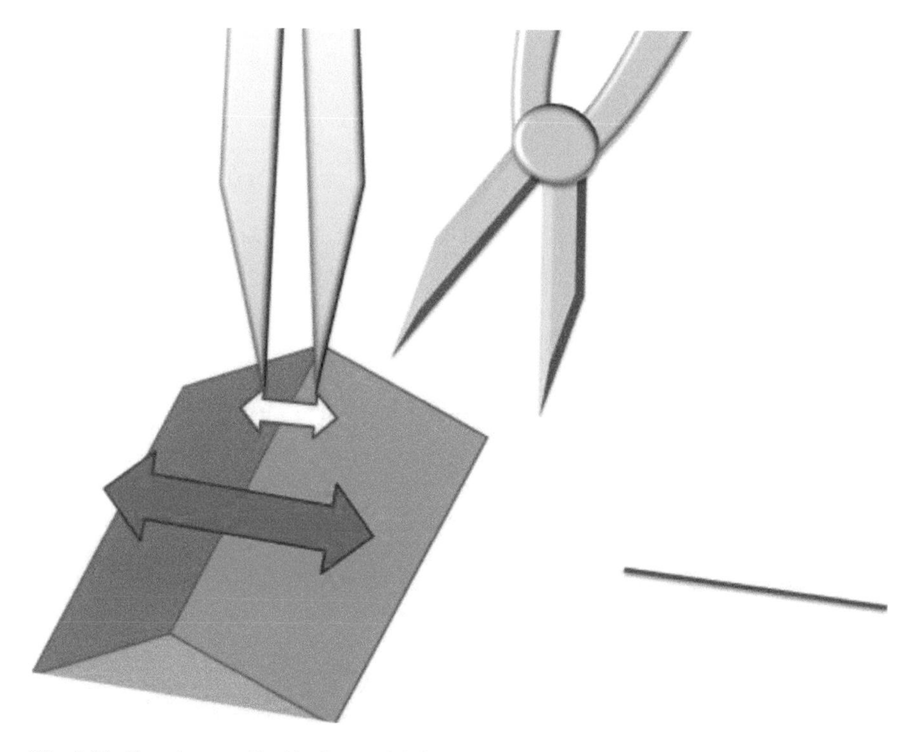

Fig. 4.24 Grasping a malleable tissue with forceps to allow it incision is best done parallel to the incision for a straight wound

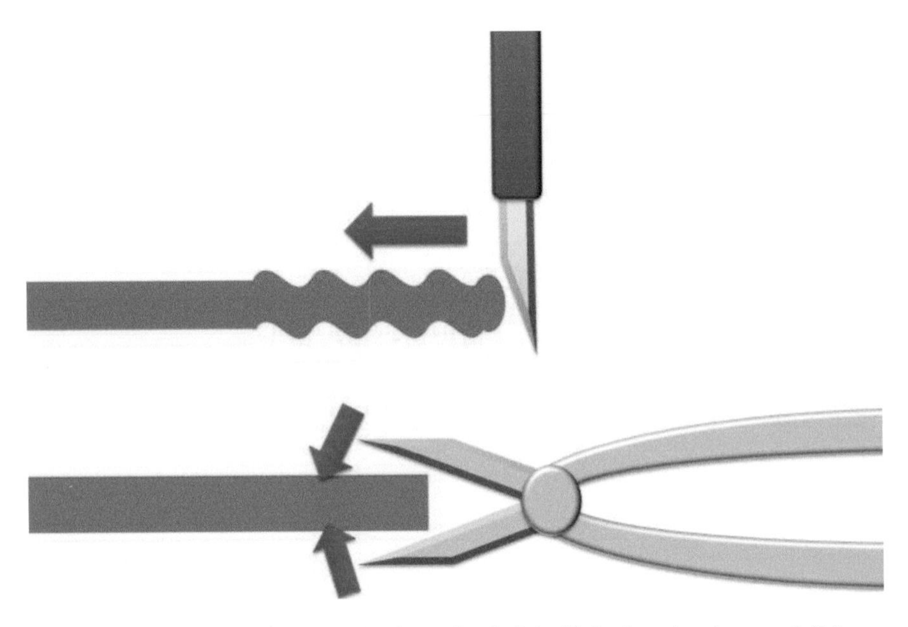

Fig. 4.25 A simple blade may push the tissue ahead of the blade distorting the wound. Scissors can be inserted to act vertically preventing the movement of the tissue

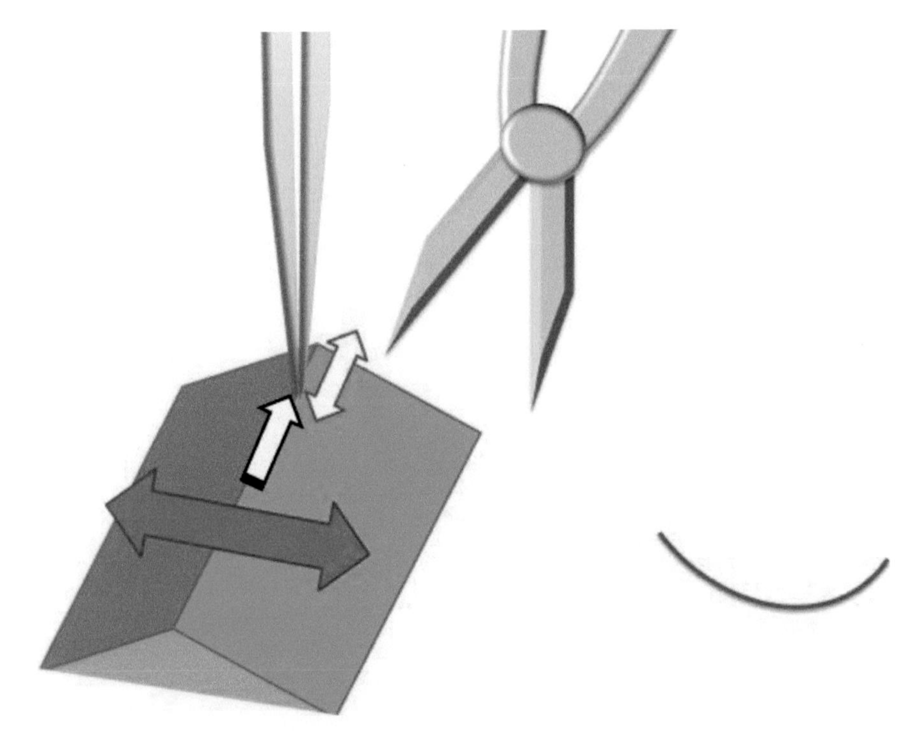

Fig. 4.26 Grasping the tissue perpendicular to the incision creates a curved wound because the tissue is compressed by the forceps

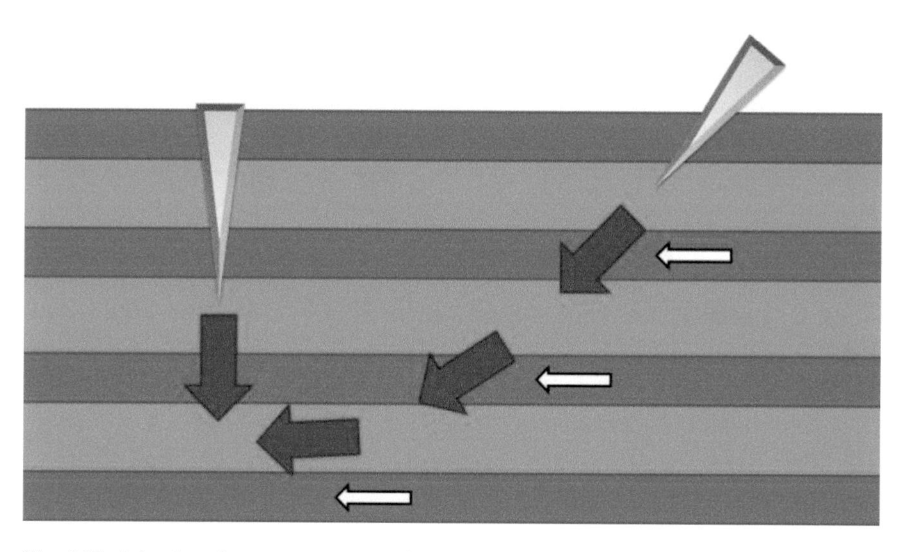

Fig. 4.27 A laminated structure acts to deflect a blade in a curved profile along one of the less resistant layers if the blade is applied at an angle

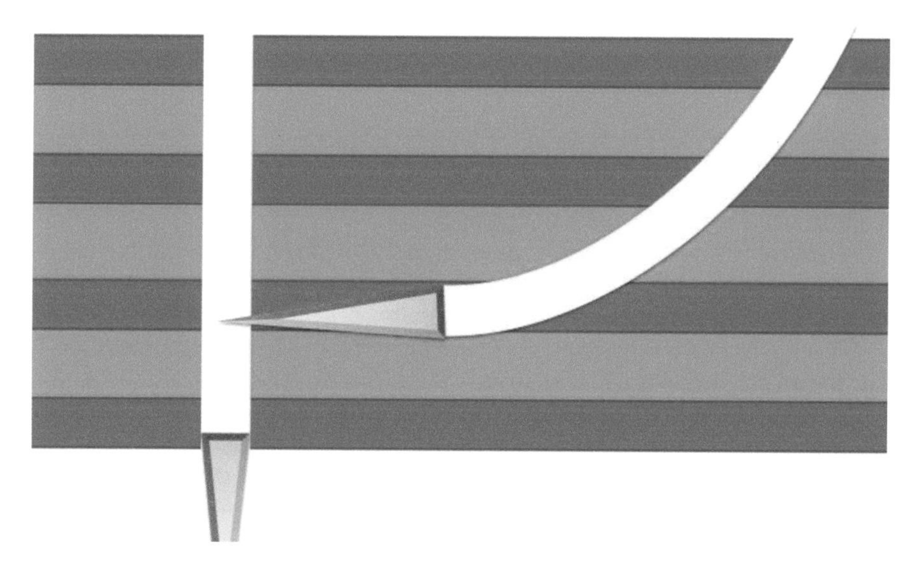

Fig. 4.28 A perpendicular incision is not deviated but an angled one is flattened off

In a soft structure the orifice created by a round bodied needle will naturally close, e.g., a hypodermic needle in the skin. Inserting a round body needle through a rigid structure creates a circular orifice, which will stay open after removal of the needle. Inserting a round-bodied instrument through a flat incision we will distort the incision risking leakage of fluid.

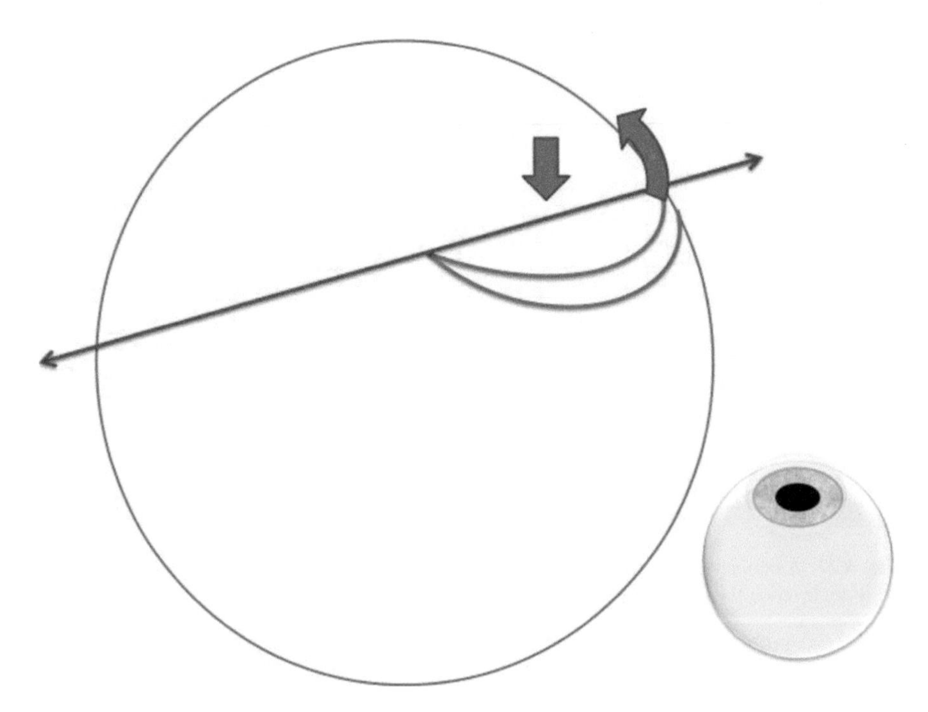

Fig. 4.29 In a spherical object the wound when elevated rotates around a line between the end of the would

If the cylindrical instrument is twisted perpendicular to the wound the effect of the distortion is increased. In a similar fashion if a force is applied to the instrument to the wound edge the wound is further opened 4.

It is easier often to commence insertion of a cylindrical instrument through a straight wound by applying the instrument at an angle so that the curve of the circular end of the instrument can be used to gradually open up the wound.

Rotating the instrument sideways in the wound can be used as a temporary measure to seal the wound (Figs. 4.33, 4.34, 4.35, 4.36, 4.37, 4.38, 4.39, and 4.40).

As we have seen sloped, tangential wounds are often used in the globe. The angle of the slope can be varied but the curvature of the eye must be considered. If the angle is too shallow there is a risk that the incision will not enter the eye. Even if the eye is entered, the long track of the incision risks injury to delicate intraocular structures. A steeper incision however risks creating a wound, which is less stable. Therefore a short wound is hard to seal but has a low chance of tissue injury whereas a long wound is easy to seal but has a high chance of tissue injury. In fact an angled wound may have a curved profile and not a straight one because of its interaction with the tissue during its creation. Be careful about rotating and instrument with in the tissue to increase the angle, because this may tear the tissue internally and any structures within. Therefore any change in angulation of an instrument while still in the tissue should be kept to a minimum (Figs. 4.41, 4.42, 4.43, 4.44, 4.45, 4.46, 4.47, 4.48, 4.49, and 4.50).

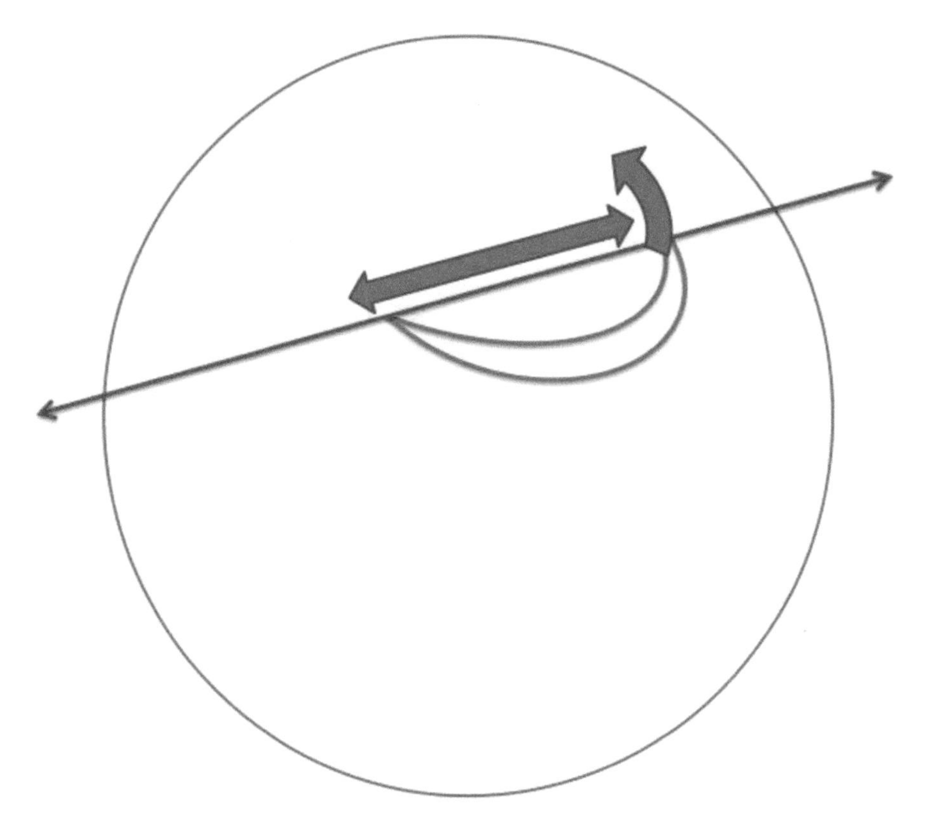

Fig. 4.30 At the line the tissue is depressed and straightened by the elevation of the wound

FEA

Surgeons aim to achieve self-sealing wounds through constructing long incisions. Long incisions are constructed by passing the blade at a tangent to the curvature of the globe. Regardless of the design of blades, static friction will always be generated at the contact point between the blade tip and the tissue prior to scleral penetration. The generated friction load will lead to the displacement of the eyeball in the direction of the load and also leads to deformational strain in the tissue. Surgeons usually attempt to minimise the displacement by stabilising the eyeball using another tool (usually toothed forceps) applied on the surface on the opposite side of the eyeball hemisphere. While it is true that stabilising the eyeball in this manner effectively reduces or stops eyeball displacement, it also increases the deformational strain generated in eyeball as the latter becomes compressed between the blade and the stabilising tool. Deformational strain in the eyeball results in various degrees of indentation and change in the angle at which the blade penetrates the tissue leading to a change the length of the incision. Adequate angulation of the incisions is important in the construction of self-sealing wound.

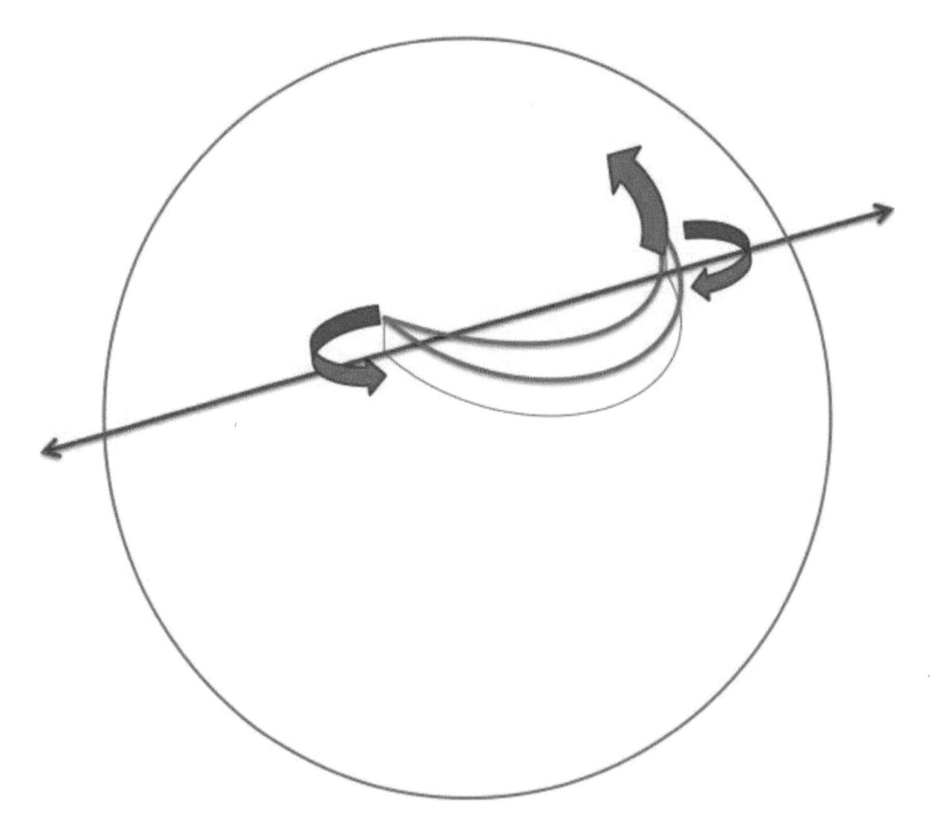

Fig. 4.31 If the wound has depth, the wound profile and the ends of the wound undergoes tortional forces

Finite element analysis of sclera shows that the location at which the surgeon stabilises the sclera, has a striking effect on the length of scleral incision. Due to the generated deformational strain, the length of the incision is shortest when the stabilising tool is placed on the area that corresponds to the entry site but on the opposite half of the hemisphere i.e., when the peak of the scleral dome lays midpoint between the entry site and the stabilised area. Moving the stabilising tool closer to the entry site or further away from entry site can help in constructing longer incisions. When the stabilising tool is applied at locations closer to the entry site and the stabilising tool is applied perpendicular to the blade plane there is a risk of slippage of the stabilising tool. Stabilising further away from the wound helps the tool to be angled away from the perpendicular (Fig. 4.51).

When creating a flap in a lamellar tissue there are strands of attachments between the lamellae. In order to maintain a constant depth of flap it is useful to put these fibres on stretch which exposes them for easy incision. This aids remaining within a lamellar plane at particular depth. By bending the flap over on itself only a few strands are exposed to cut. This can be used to minimise the length of each incision. In contrast by keeping the flap more perpendicular more fibres are exposed for each cut increasing the length of each incision.

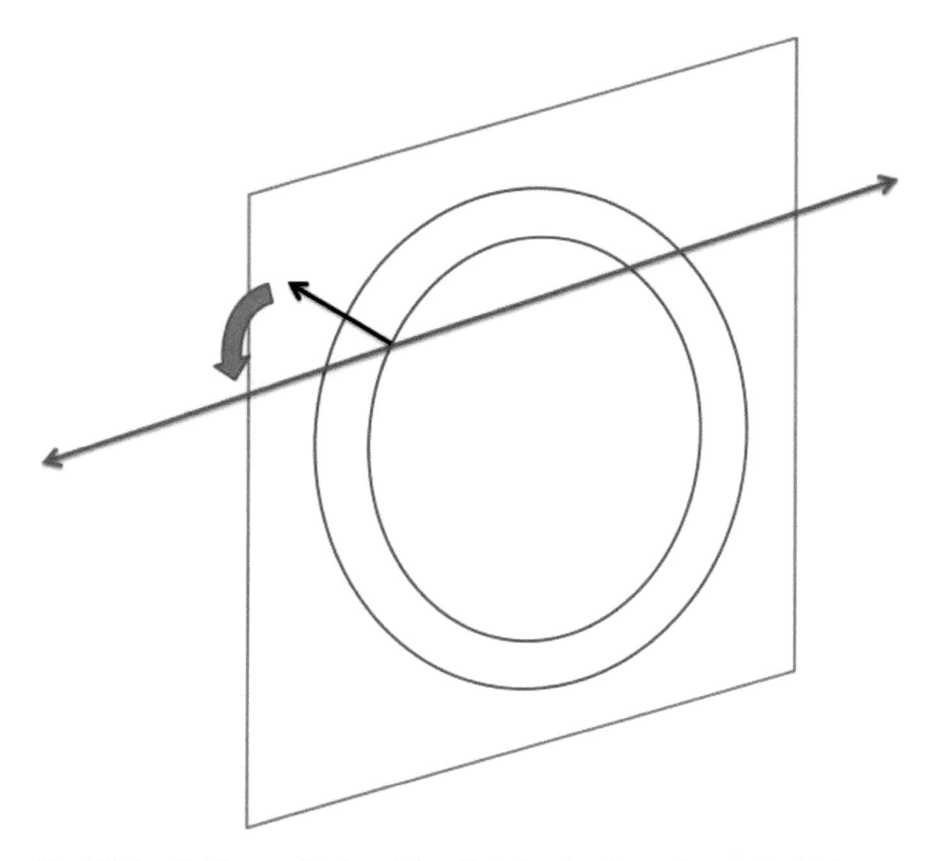

Fig. 4.32 In effect the wound in its radial profile is forced to flatten along the line joining the interior ends of the wound of when the wound is elevated

The flap can be made thicker and thinner by adjusting where the fibres are cut. This provides precise control over the depth of the incision. This can be achieved by adjusting the vertical depth of the blade, or when the flap is folded upon itself by incising closer to the flap or closer to the basal layer (Figs. 4.52, 4.53, 4.54, and 4.55).

In some circumstances tissues are manipulated without the use of blades, for example the removal of membranes from the surfaces of tissues. Often membranes have pegs of attachment to the underlying layer and not a diffuse attachment. The optimum angle for applying force to the pegs of attachment rather than to the membrane the underlying tissue has been calculated at 140°, that is the membrane folded over itself and pulled tangentially. A peg of attachment can be manipulated by pulling the membrane in different directions around the peg to finally release its adhesion (Fig. 4.56).

Some tissues are torn rather than cut. These tissues usually have an inherent stiffness, which makes some amenable to a controlled tear. In any tissue such as this a small slit in the tissue can leave the tissue vulnerable to an uncontrolled rip. For a circular incision made in this way, an irregularity in the circle, which points into the centre of the circle, we will be stable. However, an irregularity, which points to the outside of the circle, we will be vulnerable to tear externally (Figs. 4.57 and 4.58).

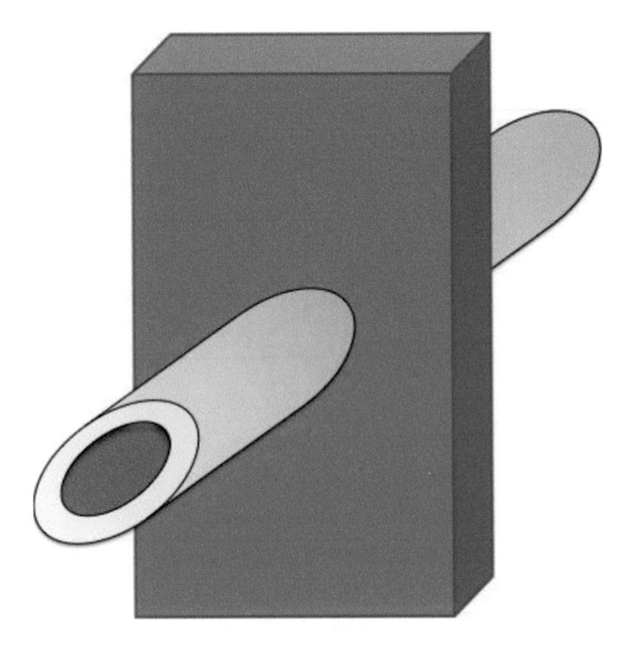

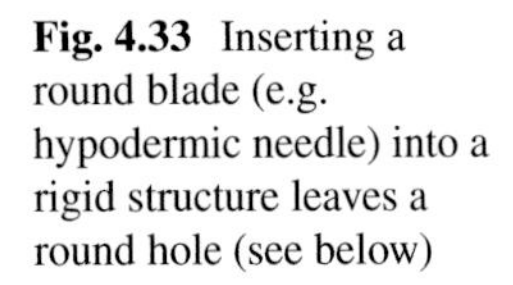

Fig. 4.33 Inserting a round blade (e.g. hypodermic needle) into a rigid structure leaves a round hole (see below)

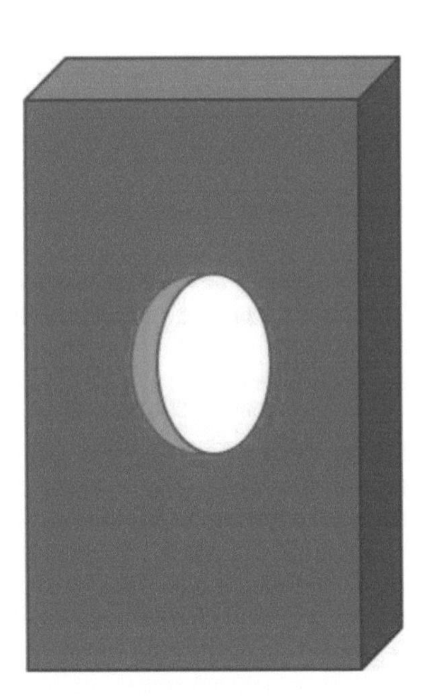

Fig. 4.34 This can be difficult to seal

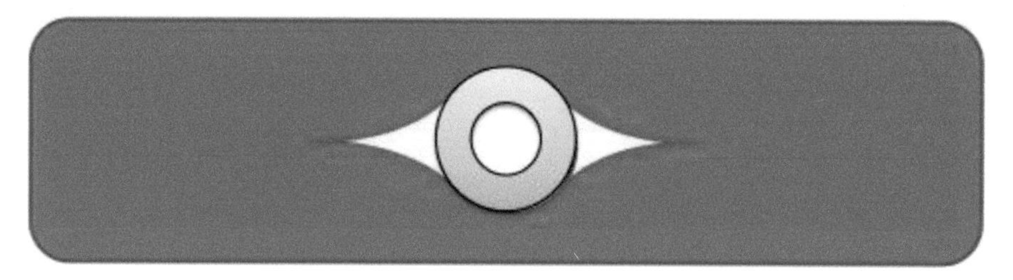

Fig. 4.35 Inserting a cylindrical instrument into a flat wound opens up the wound as shown risking leakage

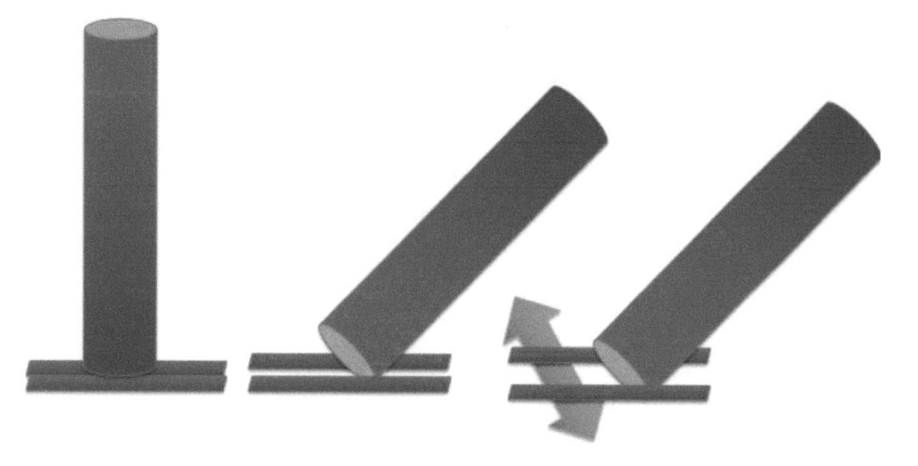

Fig. 4.36 Presenting a cylindrical instrument to a slit wound at an angle helps insertion and the curve of the instrument can be used to gradually open the wound

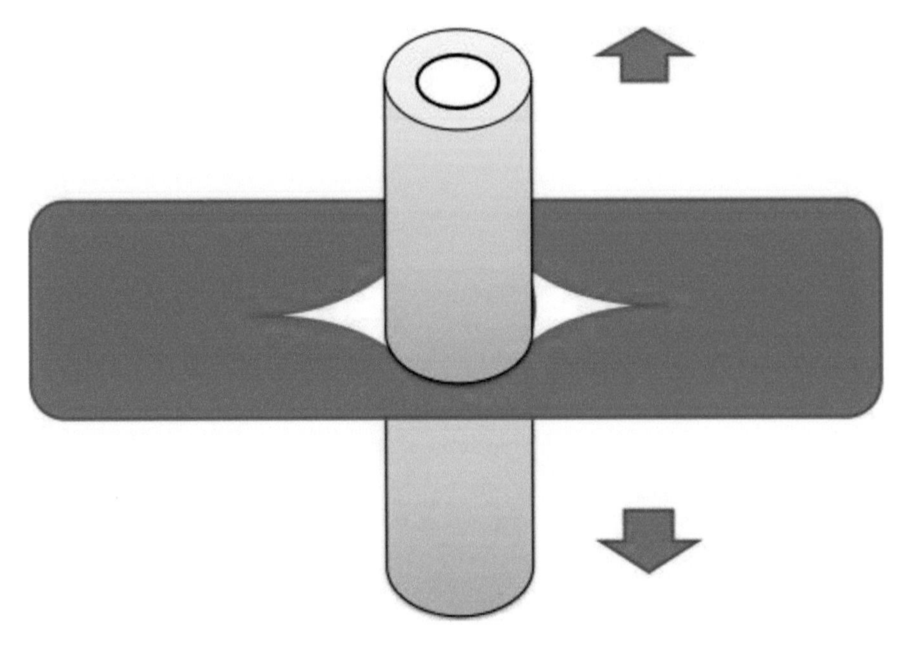

Fig. 4.37 Any twisting or distortion of the instrument opens the cavity further

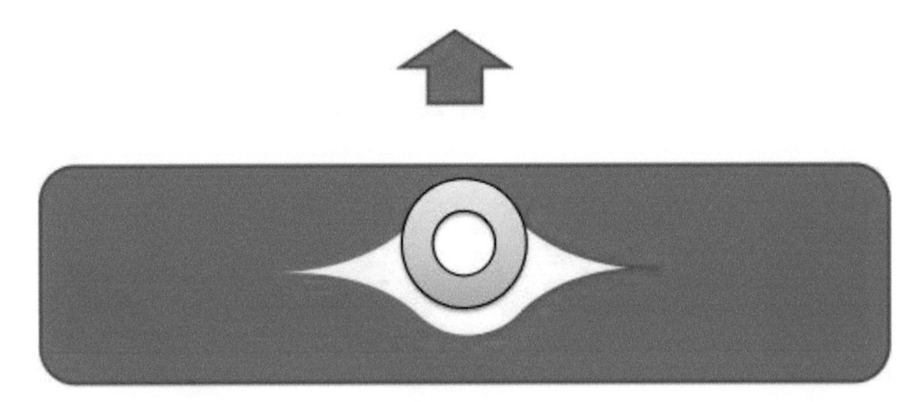

Fig. 4.38 Pressure from the instrument perpendicular to the wound will open the wound

FEA, Continuous Curvilinear Capsulorhexis and the Surgical Plane

In order to construct a round continuous curvilinear capsulorhexis, the surgeon must take into consideration the orientation of the anterior capsule plane. Failure to do so may result in an unexpected oval shaped capsulorhexis instead of a round one (Fig. 4.58). Oval shaped capsulotomies may result in partial capsular overlap with anterior and posterior capsule fusion and anterior displacement of the IOL and myopic shift. Clearly, these results are problematic, especially with a multifocal lens (Fig. 4.59).

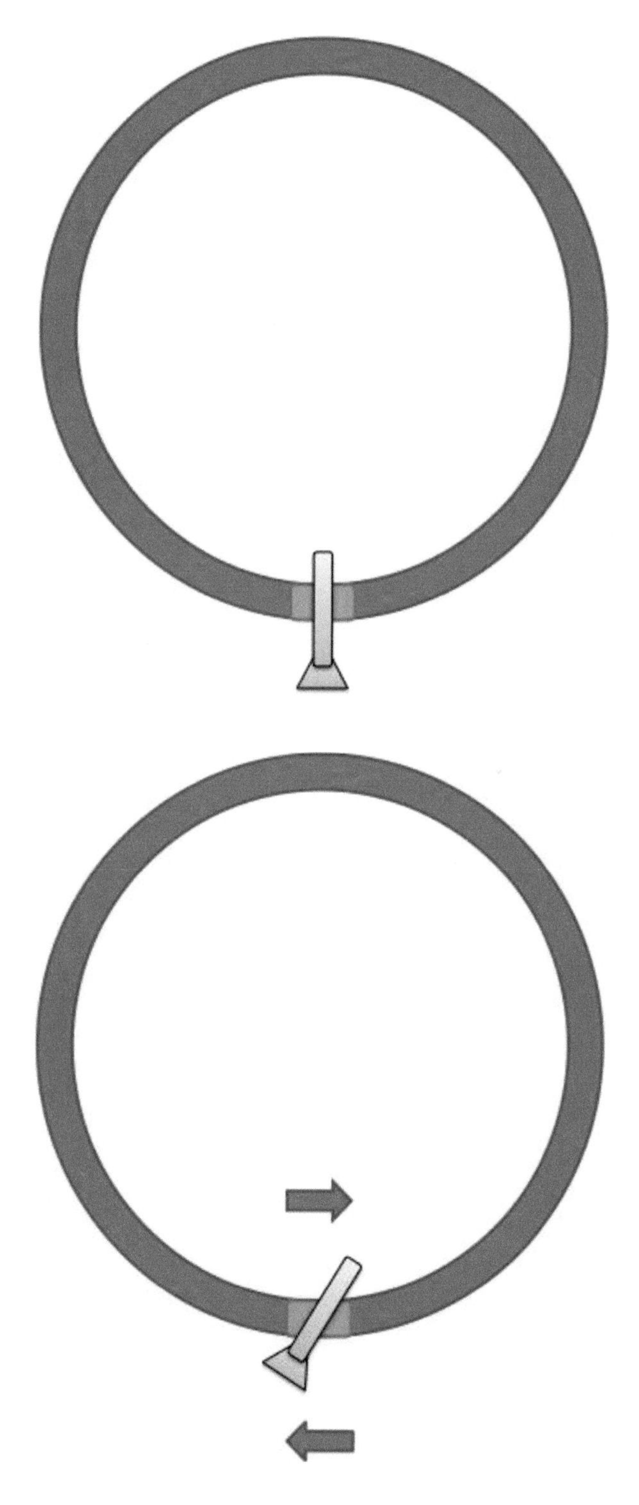

Fig. 4.39 An instrument can be angled to temporarily close an wound and reduce leakage, see below

Fig. 4.40 See Fig. 4.39

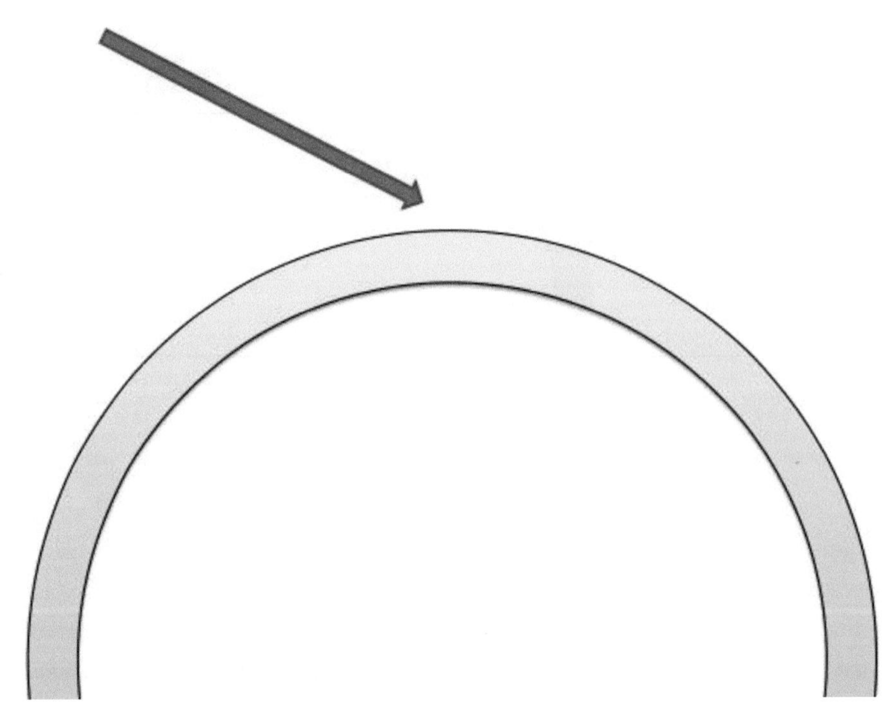

Fig. 4.41 If the angle of insertion is too narrow there is a risk that the blade not to penetrate the eye, see below

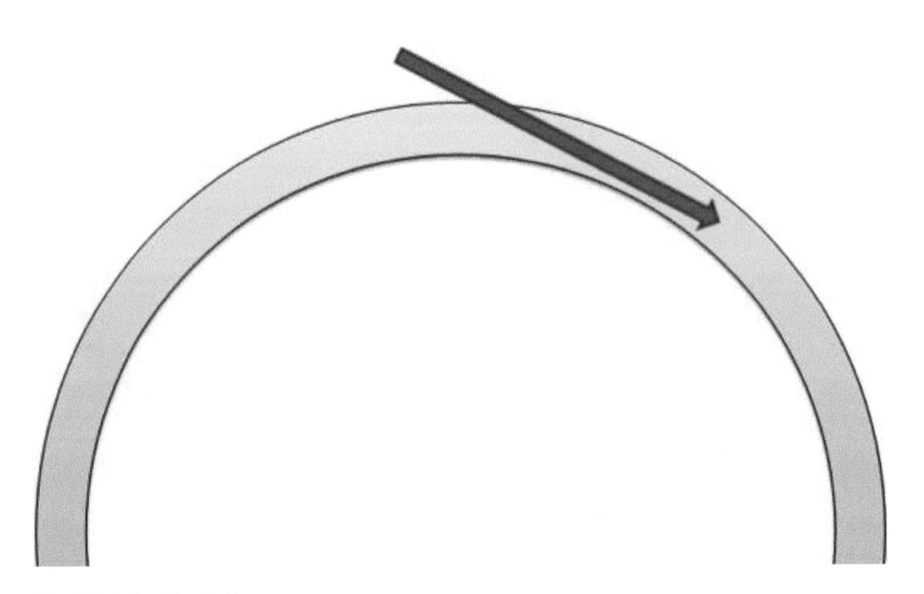

Fig. 4.42 See Fig. 4.41

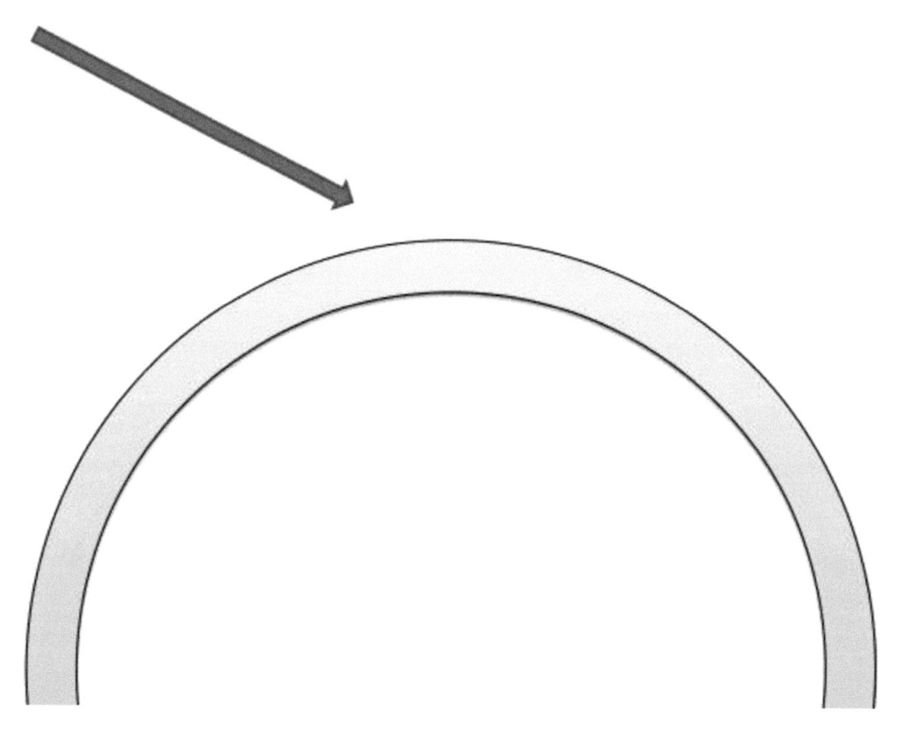

Fig. 4.43 Care has been taken to avoid damage to the internal curvature of the structure by inserting the instrument too far, see below

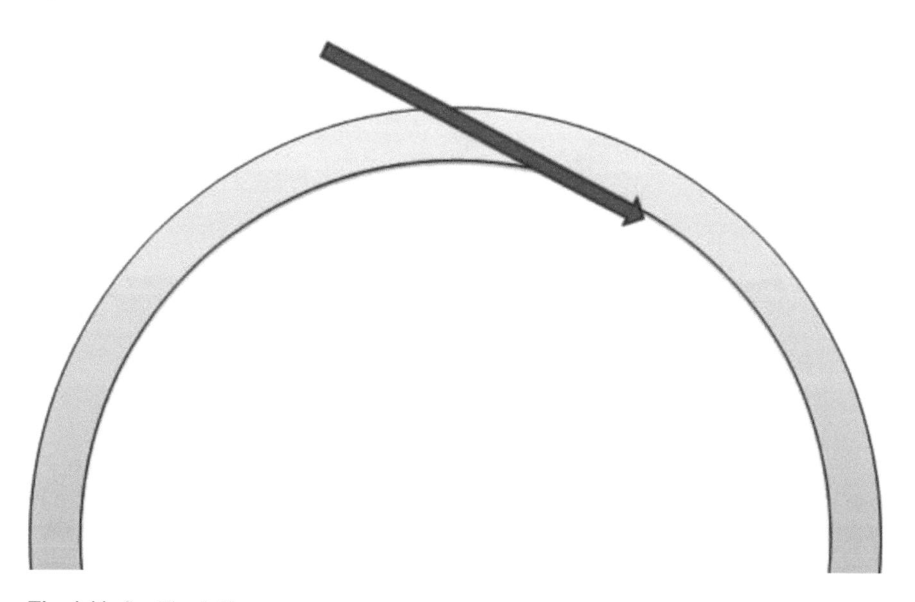

Fig. 4.44 See Fig. 4.43

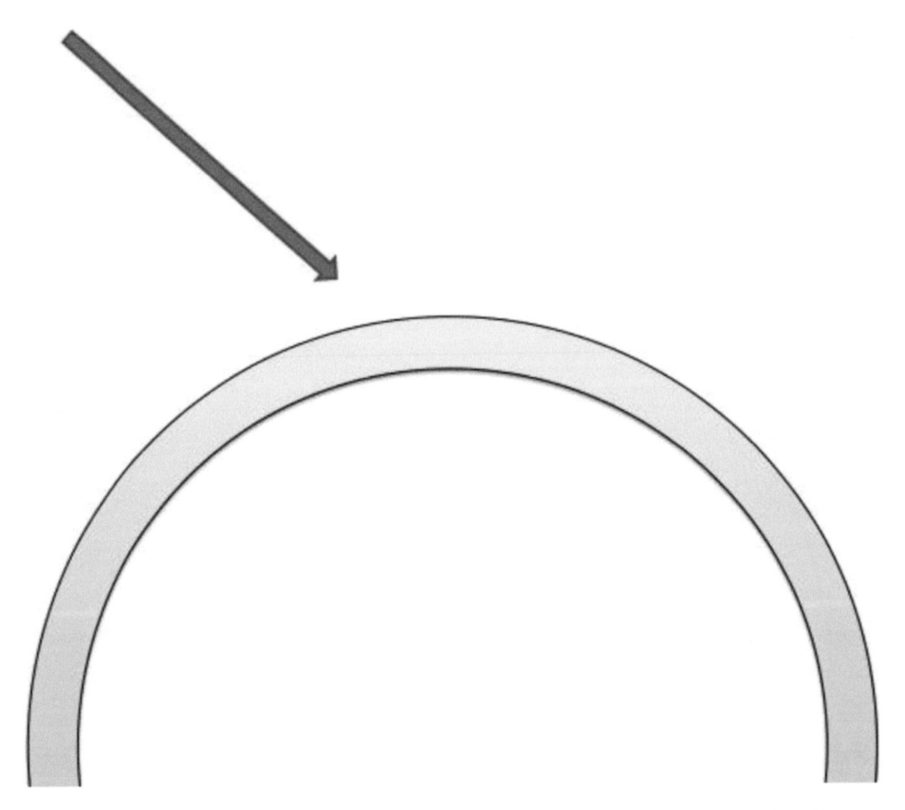

Fig. 4.45 A steeper insertion avoids internal injury but leads to a shortened wound less likely to self seal, see below

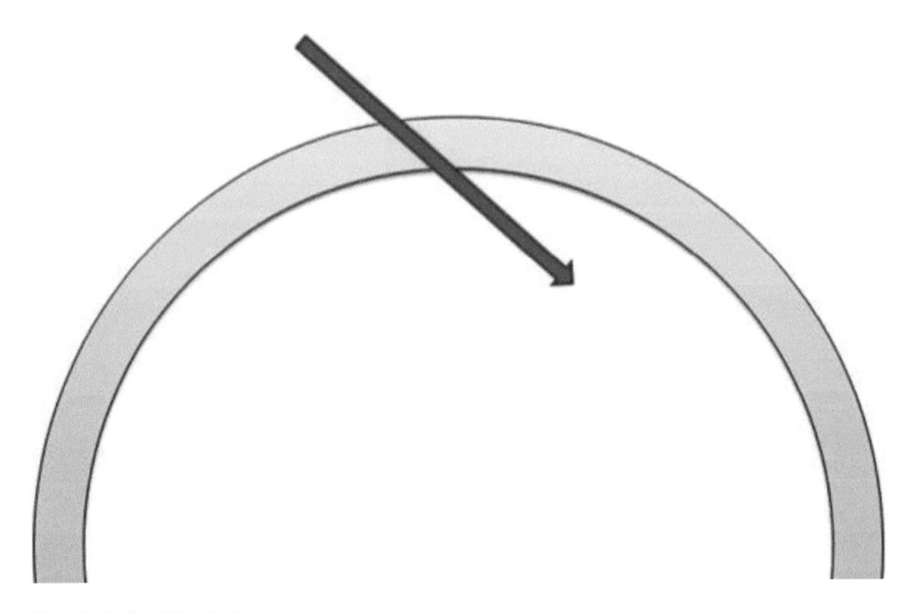

Fig. 4.46 See Fig. 4.44

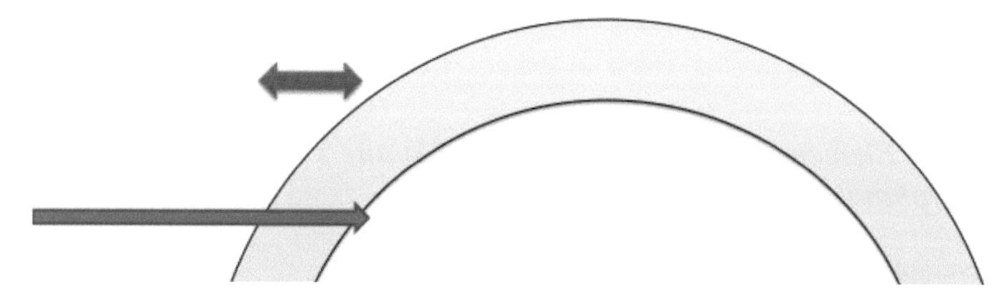

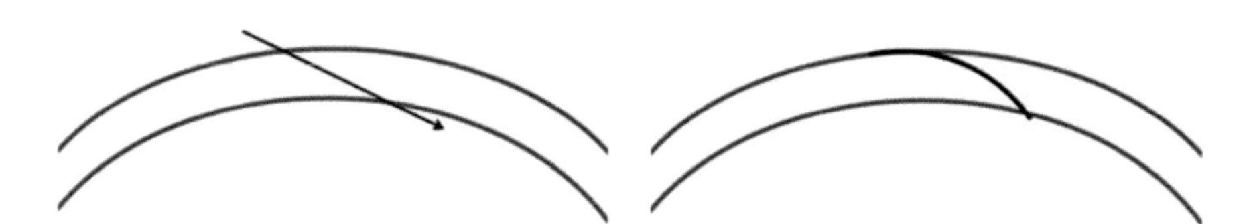

Fig. 4.47 The short wound reduces risk of injury but increases the chance of instability

Fig. 4.48 We may think we are going to created a straight wound but could, in fact, be creating a curved one because of movement of the tissue

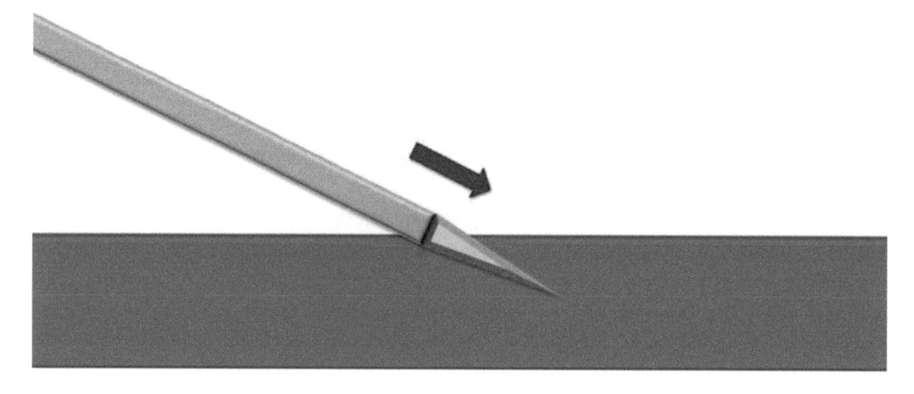

Fig. 4.49 Rotating a blade within the structure can tear the tissue, see below

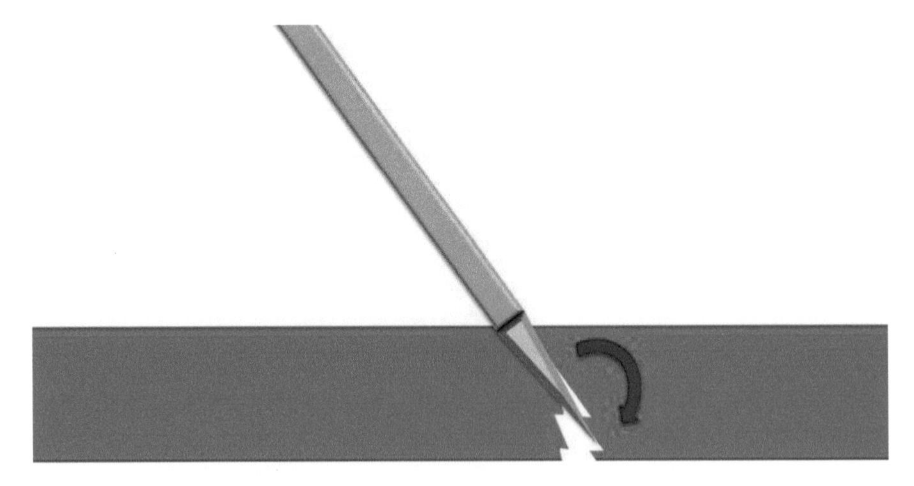

Fig. 4.50 See Fig. 4.49

Finite Element Analysis Application of Young's Modulus in Ophthalmic Surgery

Example 1 – Lens Capsule Versus Lens Cortex

When attempting to start capsulorhexis, sometimes the surgeon may inadvertently engage some lens cortex material into the tip of his capsulorhexis forceps. In such circumstances the forceps-tissue contact surface area will be shared between the cortex material and the lens capsule and consequently reduces friction and weakens the bond between the forceps and capsule. Furthermore because the Young's modulus of the lens is 364 times higher than the cortex material (i.e.: the capsule is stiffer) [1], the amount of the stress generated in the capsule will be 98 times higher than that in the cortex, therefore it will be more likely for the capsule to retract back and slip from the forceps tip before the cortex Fig. 4.2. If the surgeon is unwary of this he or she may continue pulling the cortex and wonder why his or her capsulorhexis is ineffective, particularly because the grasping tip of the forceps usually falls in the blind spot of the surgeon. Refer to chapter forceps to read about the blind spot of intraocular forceps (Fig. 4.60).

Example 2 – Internal Limiting Membrane Versus Vitreous Cortex

Another example is where there is a thin schitic layer of vitreous over the internal limiting membrane. In such circumstances when the surgeon tries to grasp the internal limiting membrane with intraocular forceps, a large amount of vitreous will compete with the internal limiting membrane over the small surface area at the grasping tip of the forceps. Internal limiting membrane is 50 times stiffer than the vitreous and consequently the stress generated at the internal limiting membrane is

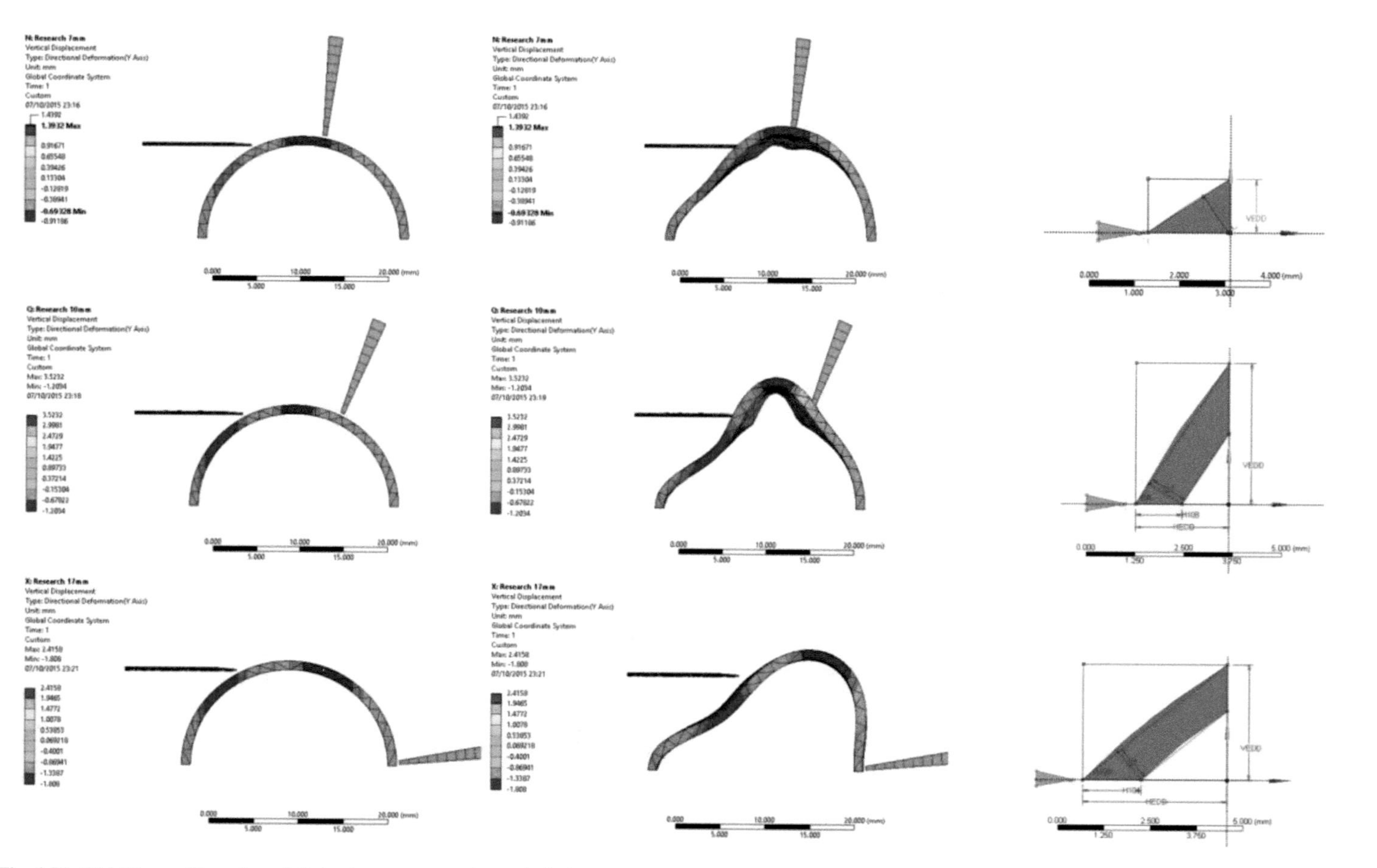

Fig. 4.51 FEA The position of a stabilising instrument on the eyeball alters angle of slope of the incision. If the instrument is close or far away form the incision a better slope is created. Due distortion of the globe, a fixation point at medium distance can create a steeper slope and prevent adequate shelving of the wound

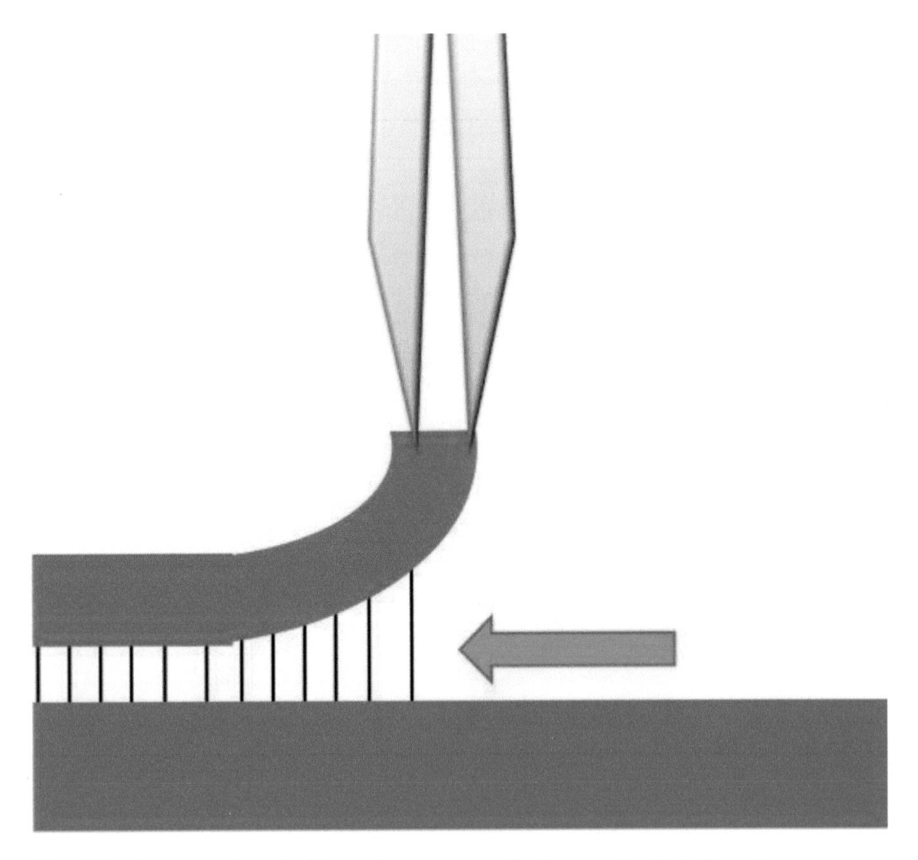

Fig. 4.52 Elevating a flap of a fibrous tissue presents the fibres to the blade for cutting

41 times higher than the vitreous. Therefore it is more likely for the internal limiting membrane to retract back and slip from the tip of the forceps before the vitreous. The unwary surgeon may not realise this, particularly because the vitreous is transparent and he or she may attempt to grasp deeper in the tissue, running the risk of iatrogenic retinal breaks (Fig. 4.61).

FEA Continuous Circular Capsulorhexis and Capsular Fold Configurations

A well performed continuous circular capsulorhexis facilitates smooth circular capsular opening of different sizes, and produces a strong capsular rim that resists tearing even when stretched during lens material removal or lens implantation [2]. It is not possible to describe adequately the vectors that must be applied to complete the

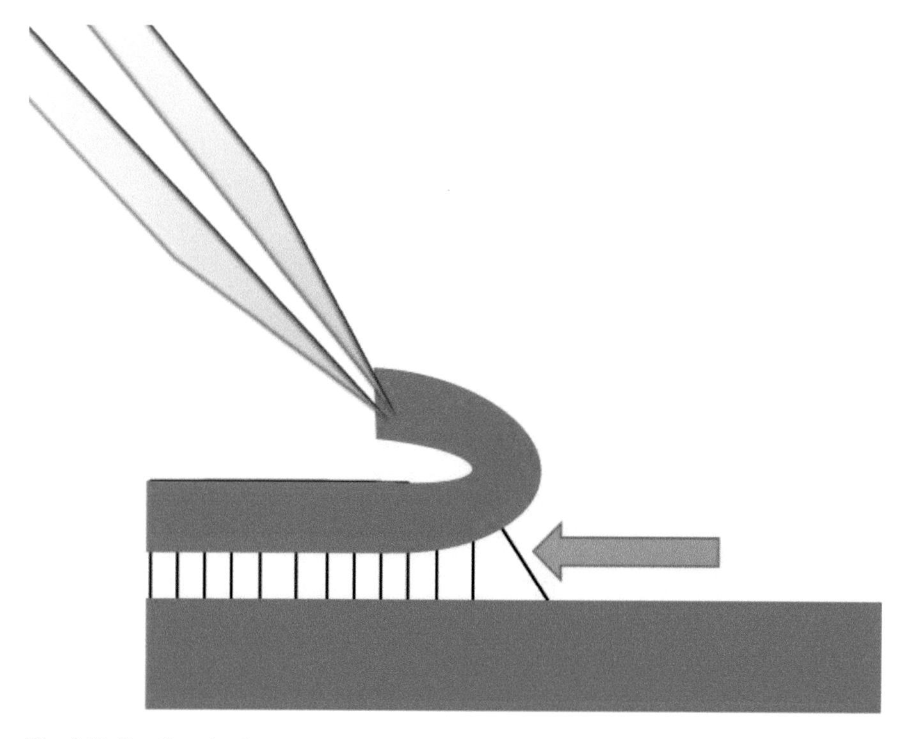

Fig. 4.53 Bending the flap over upon itself reduces the number of fibres that can be cut in one sweep

capsulorhexis. However some prediction could be made by carefully observing the capsular fold configuration. The following configurations could be recognised when capsulorhexis is carried out.

Zero Fold Configuration

This configuration arises when the flap is pulled forward away from its origin. Because the flap is not pulled backward upon itself, no fold is formed and therefore called "Zero Fold Configuration". When the capsule is pulled in this way the generated stress lines in the capsules will be directed sharply to the centre of the lens. This is a very efficient way of steering capsulorhexis margin into the centre of the lens for the reason that it leads to a sharp inward turn. It is usually used to rescue an extending capsulorhexis but not as primary method of capsulorhexis as it is likely to result in small capsulorhexis. It must be noted that this type of configuration can put high tension on the zonules and it should not be use as a rescue method if the surgeon suspects extensions that have already reached the zonules. In such cases the surgeon may prefer to use scissors to start capsulorhexis from the opposite direction or convert it to can opener method.

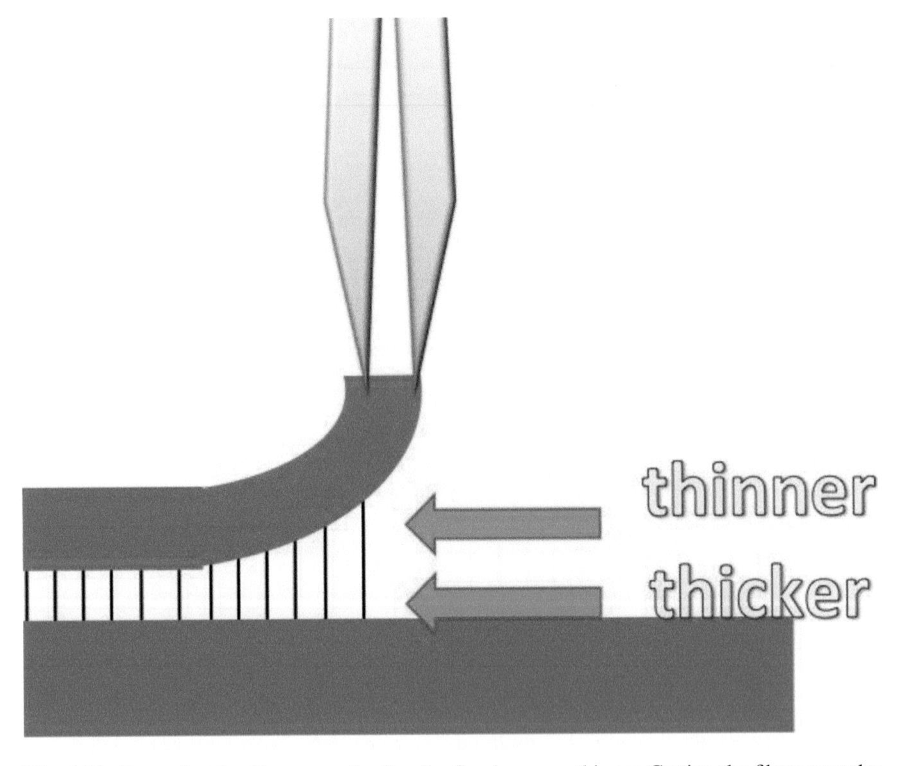

Fig. 4.54 By cutting the fibres near the flap the flap becomes thinner. Cutting the fibres near the base thickens the flap

Single Fold Configuration

This configuration arises when the flap is pulled backward over itself. Because the flap is pulled upon itself, a single fold is formed and therefore called "Single Fold Configuration". When the capsule is pulled in this way the generated stress lines in the capsules will be directed in a concentric pattern and parallel to the equator of the lens. Therefore this configuration is ideal to achieve an adequate sized capsulorhexis. The limitation of single fold configuration is that it is difficult to maintain its structure when the capsulorhexis is carried out on the proximal 1/3 of the lens because of the restrictions on the movement of the forceps/cystotome under within the corneal section.

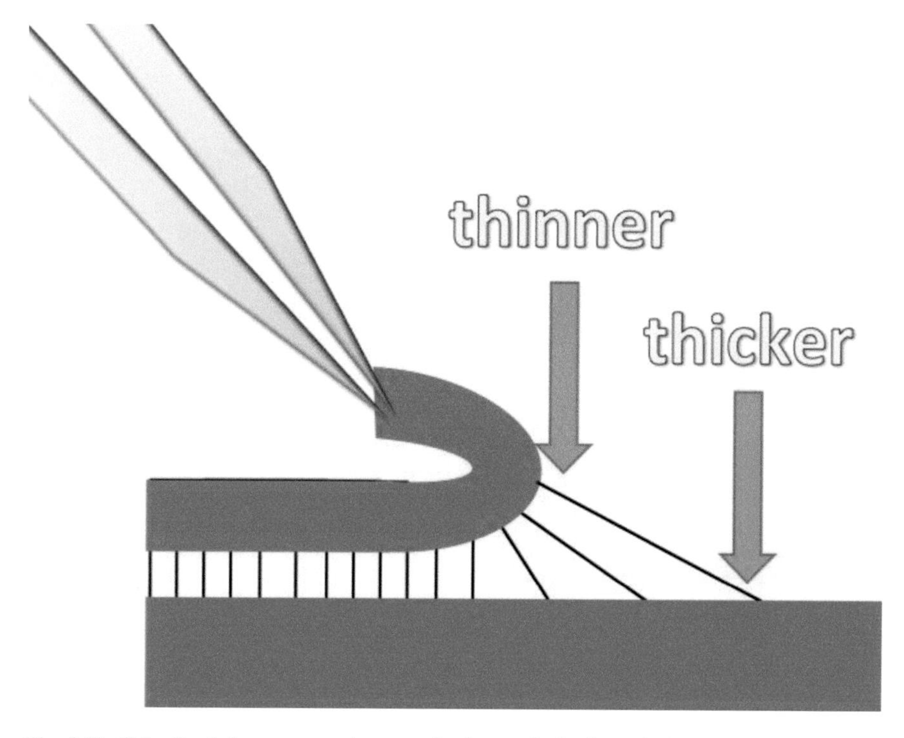

Fig. 4.55 If the flap is bent over cutting near the flap on the horizontal plane makes the flap thinner, whereas cutting further away from the flap thickens the flap

Double Fold Configuration

Double fold configuration forms when a large flap is pulled within the limited boundaries of the anterior chamber. This configuration usually arises when capsulorhexis is carried out on the proximal 1/3 of the lens. The limitation of double fold configuration is the tendency of the capsulorhexis to extend to the zonules if the surgeon is not careful (Fig. 4.62).

FEA Capsulorhexis Size and Nucleus Rotation

After adequate hydrodissection the surgeon usually attempts to rotate the nucleus within the capsule. Increased friction between the nucleus and the capsule results in higher shear stress at the capsule when nucleus rotation is attempted.

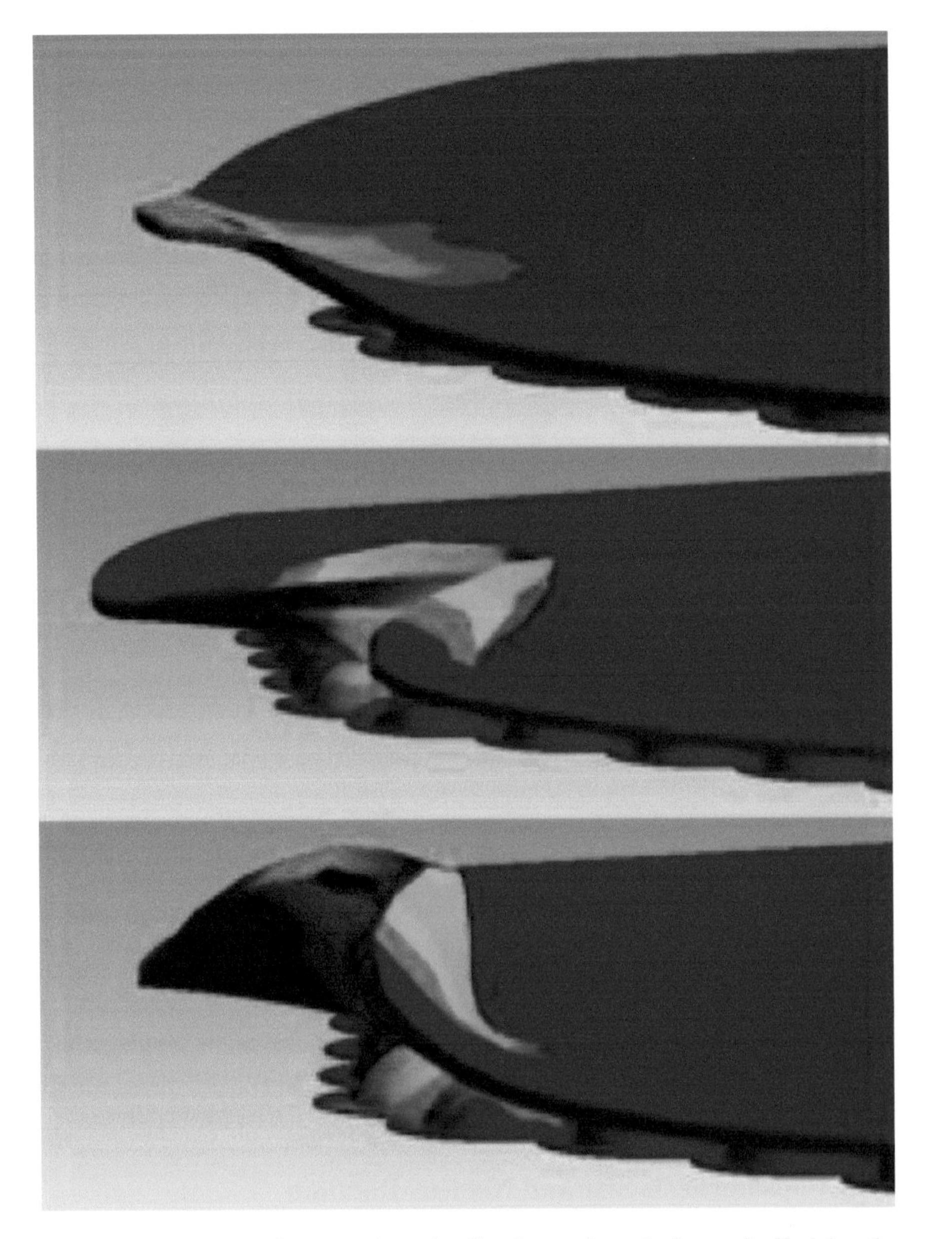

Fig. 4.56 FEA When peeling a membrane bending the membrane back upon itself minises the stress on the membrane and underlying structure and maximises the stress on the adhesion points thereby allowing safer separation of the membrane

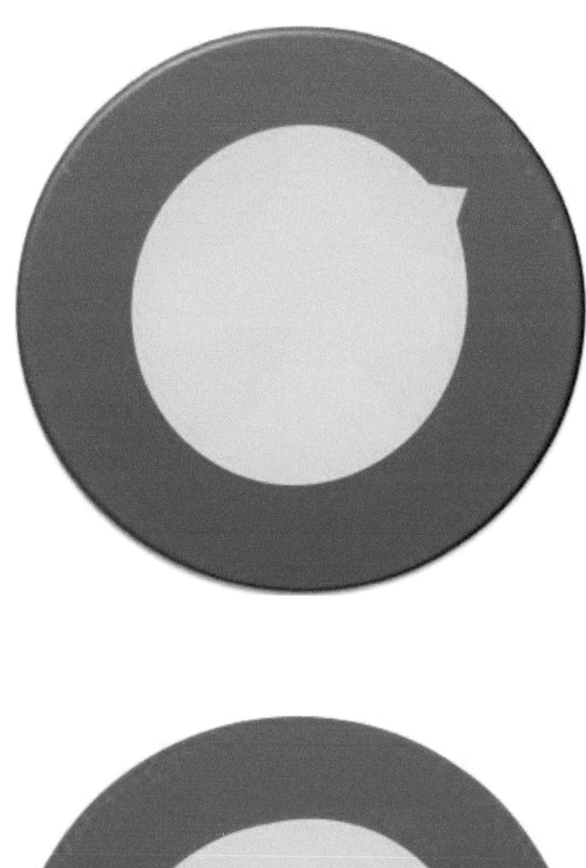

Fig. 4.57 When tearing an opening in a capsule a small "nick" pointing outwards can rip the membrane radially under tension

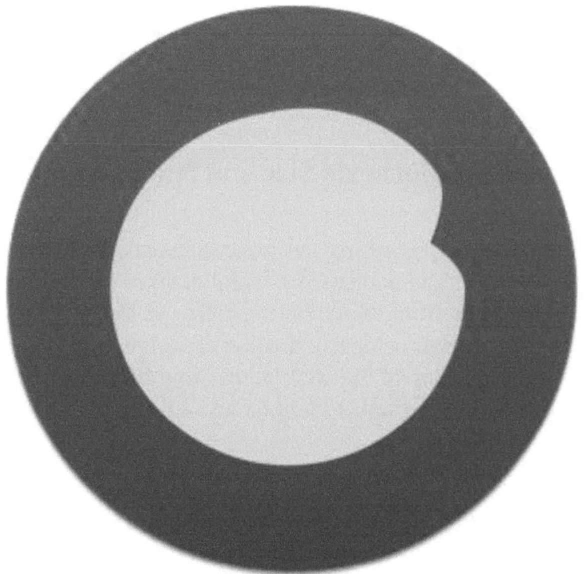

Fig. 4.58 A small inward pointing defect in the circle is stable and should not rip under tension

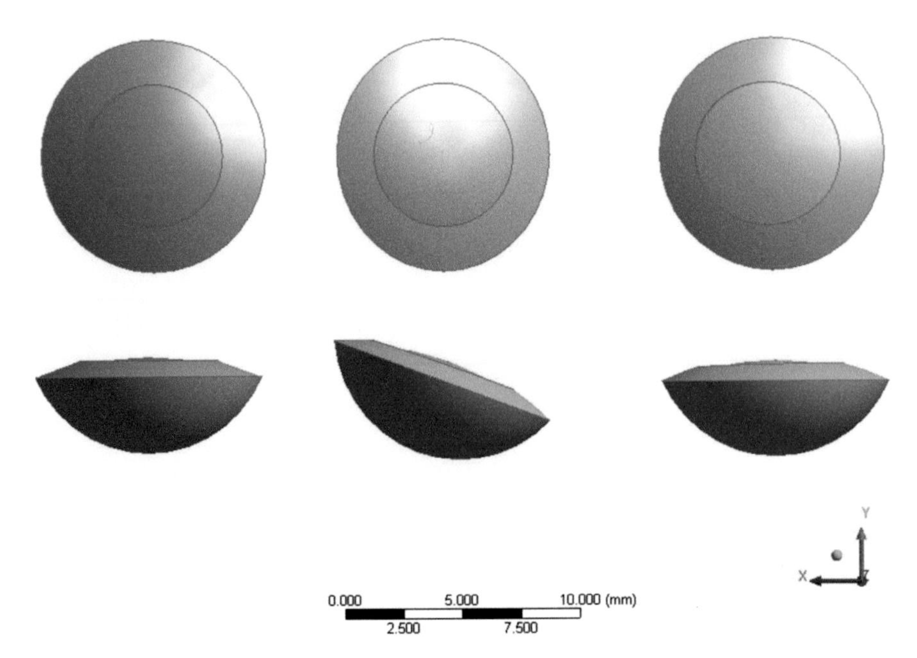

Fig. 4.59 FEA *left column* shows a round continuous curvilinear capsulorhexis (CCC) performed in a lens held in the neutral position (iris plane parallel to the floor). *Middle column* shows a presumably round CCC performed in an eye that is tilted to the right by 20° of angle. *Right column* shows the actual oval shape of the CCC created in the lens shown in the *middle column* after bringing the eye to the neutral position. *Top Row* shows the top views of the lenses as they appear under the microscope and the *bottom row* show the side views of the lenses

FEA Capsulorhexis Size and Nucleus Cracking

After adequate grooving the surgeon usually attempts to crack the nucleus within the capsule. The nucleus is usually cracked by forcing the opposing walls of the groove away from each other: resulting in the horizontal expansion of the nucleus until the crack is achieved. Smaller capsulorhexes adds more resistance on the horizontal expansion of the nucleus resulting in higher shear stress at the capsule when cracking is attempted (Figs. 4.63 and 4.64).

FEA Sculpting Central Groove and the Surgical Plane

Sculpting a central groove in the lens without taking the baseline orientation of the lens plane into account may result in a groove that is at an oblique angle to the lens plane (Fig. 8.3). This may not only result in creation of two asymmetrical halves but also makes the cracking process more challenging with higher risk of posterior capsular rupture as will be shown in the next paragraph (Fig. 4.65).

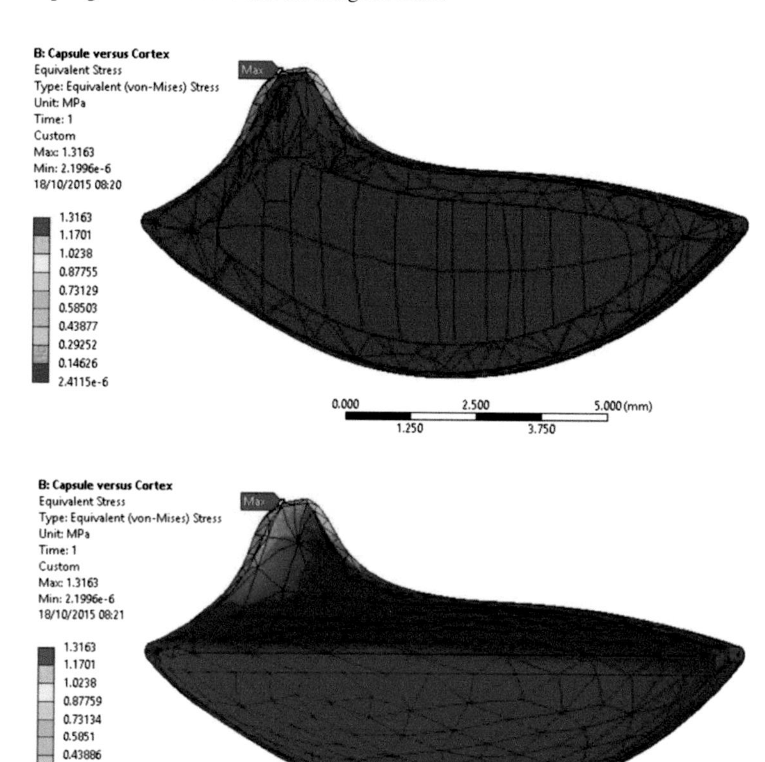

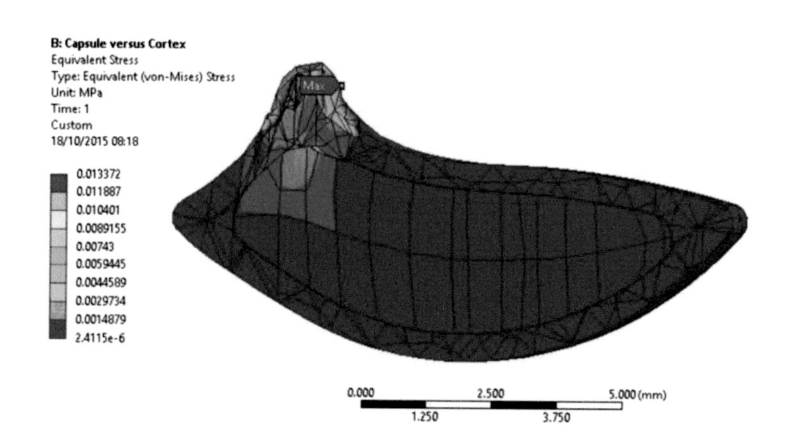

Fig. 4.60 FEA inadvertent engagement of some lens cortex material into the tip of the capsulorhexis forceps along with the capsule. Stress generated in the capsule is 98 times higher than that in the cortex, therefore it will be more likely for the capsule to retract back and slip from the forceps tip before the cortex. Top shows the capsule and the cortex engaged into the tip of the forceps, middle show the stress level in the capsule only, bottom shows stress level in the cortex and the nucleus of the lens

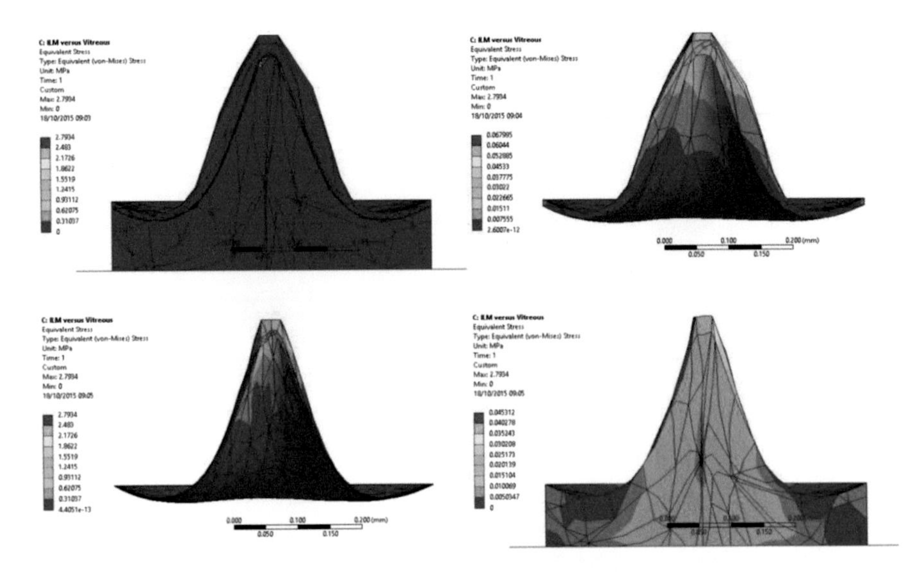

Fig. 4.61 FEA shows grasping a thin schitic layer of vitreous along with the internal limiting membrane, with the stress generated at the internal limiting membrane, which is 41 times higher than the vitreous. *Top left* shows the stress level in all layers; *top right* shows the stress level in the vitreous only; *bottom left* shows the stress level in the internal limiting membrane; *bottom right* shows the stress level at the retina only

FEA Rotation of the Nucleus and the Surgical Plane

Nucleus rotation manoeuvres are needed on many occasions during cataract surgery. Some degree of rotation is always needed after a successful curvilinear capsulorhexis and hydrodissection. Finite element analysis demonstrated that the level of shear stress generated at the edge of the anterior capsule dramatically increases when the plane of the rotational force and the plane of the lens are not correctly aligned (Fig. 4.66).

FEA Cracking the Nucleus into Quadrants and the Surgical Plane

In order to propagate a crack in the centre of a grooved lens, a horizontal force has to be applied at right angles to the side walls of the lens to displace the walls in opposite directions and for equal distance. Finite element analysis shows that when this manoeuvre is performed correctly, the nucleus/capsule shear stress ratio is greater. However, if the lens plane and/or the groove are tilted, the force may not be entirely perpendicular to the side walls, resulting in lower nucleus/capsule stress

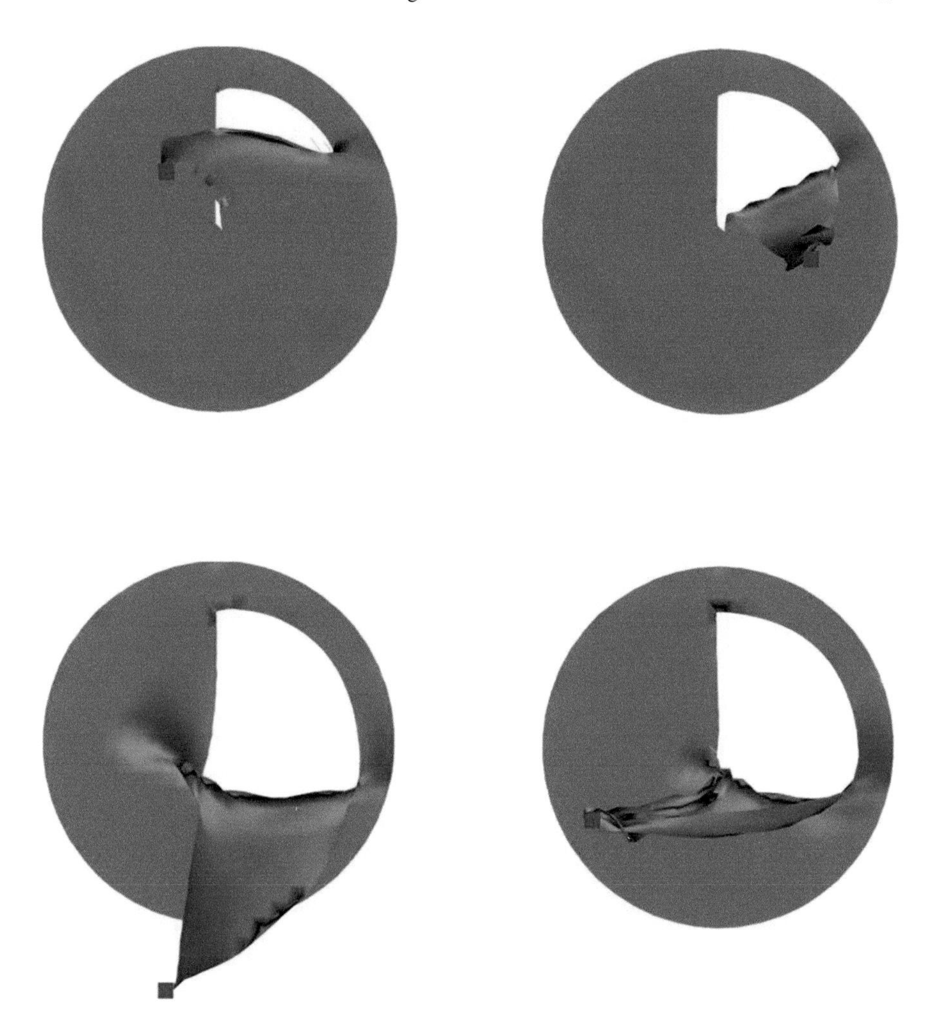

Fig. 4.62 FEA this figure shows capsulorhexis. It is not possible to describe adequately the vectors that must be applied to complete the capsulorhexis. However some prediction could be made by carefully observing the fold in the flap. *Top left* shows zero flap configuration where pulling in this direction results in a sharp inward movement of the rhexis, *Top right* shows single fold configuration, this is ideal for capsulorhexis as the rhexis will follow the direction of the pull. *Bottom left* shows the limitation of single fold as the flap grows longer. Note the forceps has to be pulled outside the boundaries of the anterior chamber to keep the integrity of single configuration on large flaps. *Bottom right*: double fold configuration that forms when a large flap is pulled within the limited boundaries of the anterior chamber. This figure emphasises the importance of regrasping the flap frequently

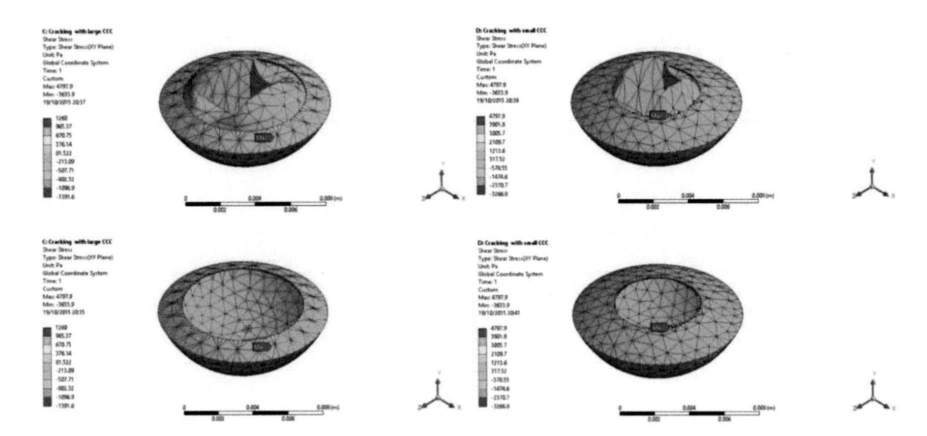

Fig. 4.63 FEA when cracking the nucleus a smaller capsulorhexis is put under more strain than a larger one

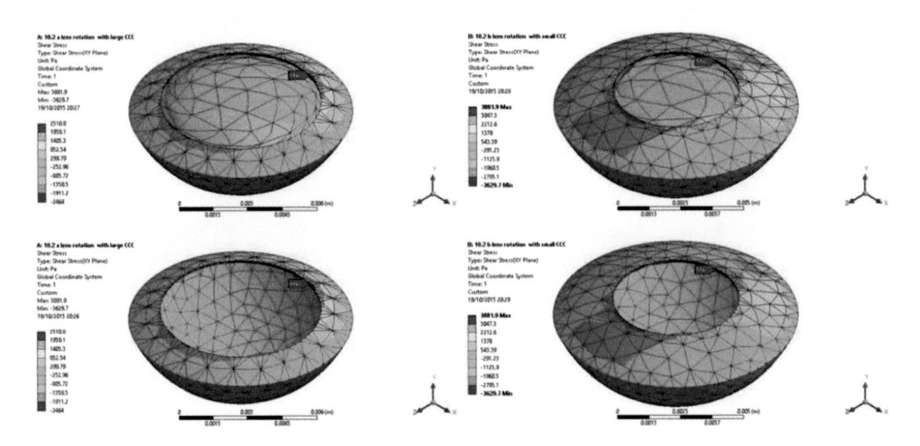

Fig. 4.64 FEA when rotating the nucleus there is more friction against the capsule when the capsultomy is small (*right column*)

levels in the nucleus and higher stress levels risking capsular damage. Force, groove, lens alignment could take one or more of the following scenarios:

Scenario 1: force is applied at right angles to the side walls of a groove that is sculpted perpendicular to the lens plane, and the lens plane is at neutral position, in such circumstances the shear stress generated at the nucleus is 0.18 of that generated in the capsule.

Scenario 2: force is applied at right angles to the side walls of a groove that is sculpted perpendicular to the lens plane, but the lens plane is tilted by 20°, in such circumstances the shear stress generated at the nucleus is 0.01 of that generated in the capsule.

Scenario 3: force is applied at right angles to the side walls of a groove that is sculpted at 20° to the lens plane, and the lens plane kept tilted by 20°, in such circumstances the shear stress generated at the nucleus is 0.02 of that generated in the capsule.

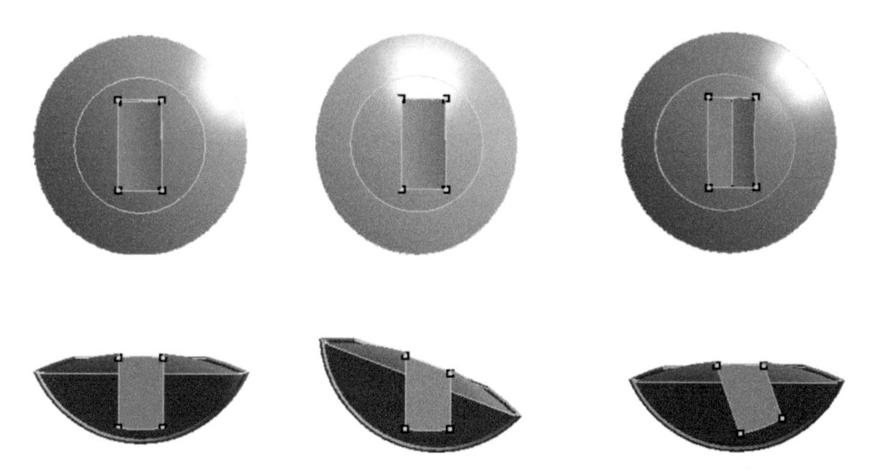

Fig. 4.65 FEA *left column* shows a central groove performed perpendicular to the lens plane in an eye that is held in the neutral position. *Middle column* shows the same groove performed carelessly in an eye that is tilted by 20° angle to the right. *Right column* shows the eye the same eye brought to the neutral position after careless grooving, now the central groove becomes at 20° angle to the microscope plane and the lens plane. *Top row* shows the top view as it appears under the microscope. *Bottom row* shows the side view of the same lenses

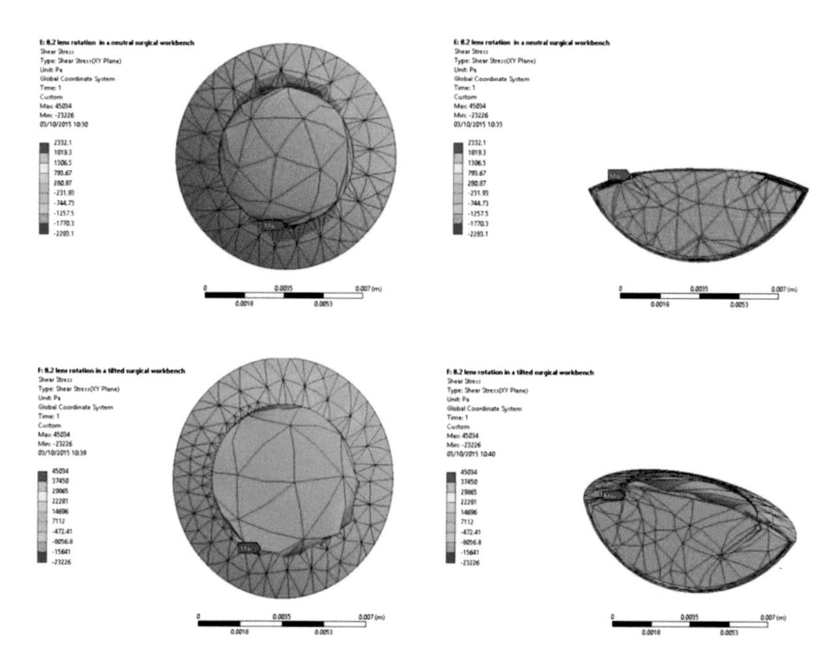

Fig. 4.66 FEA shows the shear distribution on the lens and the capsule when rotational force applied on the surface of the lens. The maximum shear force is localised at the edge of the capsule and it is 19.3 times higher when the rotational force and the lens planes are not aligned. *Top left* shows the top view of shear force distribution in a lens that is kept in the neutral position while neutral rotational force is applied to its surface. *Top right* shows the side view of shear force distribution in a lens that is kept in the neutral position while neutral rotational force is applied to its surface. *Bottom right* shows the top view of shear force distribution in a lens that is tilted by 20° while neutral rotational force is applied to its surface. *Bottom left* shows the side view of shear force distribution in a lens that is tilted by 20° while neutral rotational force is applied to its surface

Scenario 4: Imagine that the surgeon in scenario number 4 realises that he sculpted the groove at 20° angle to the plane of his lens, and he decided to bring the lens plane to neutral, in such a case the force will be applied at 20° to the side walls of a groove that is sculpted at 20° to the lens plane, with the lens plane in neutral position. In such circumstances the shear stress generated at the nucleus is 0.08 of that generated in the capsule (Table 4.1).

It must be noted that the shear stress in the capsule is higher than that of the cortex, but in the presence of a well formed curvilinear capsulorhexis the capsule becomes more tolerant to this stress, this fact highlights the importance of a completeness of the capsulorhexis. Despite this the surgeon must aim to keep the nucleus/capsule stress ratio as high as possible to achieve a safer cracking manoeuvre. Table 4.1: shows the shear stress values recorded for different scenarios. Figures show shear force distribution for different scenarios (Figs. 4.67, 4.68, 4.69, and 4.70).

Table 4.1 Shows the levels of shear stress generated in the nucleus and the capsule when cracking manoeuvre is attempted in the four circumstances mentioned above

	Shear stress level in Pa		
Scenario	Nucleus	Capsule	Nucleus/lens ratio
1	1920	10,609	0.180978
2	504.24	28,325	0.017802
3	374.73	13,842	0.027072
4	1674.3	18,965	0.088284

The ratio in scenario one has the highest ratio and should be aimed for as standard practice by the surgeon

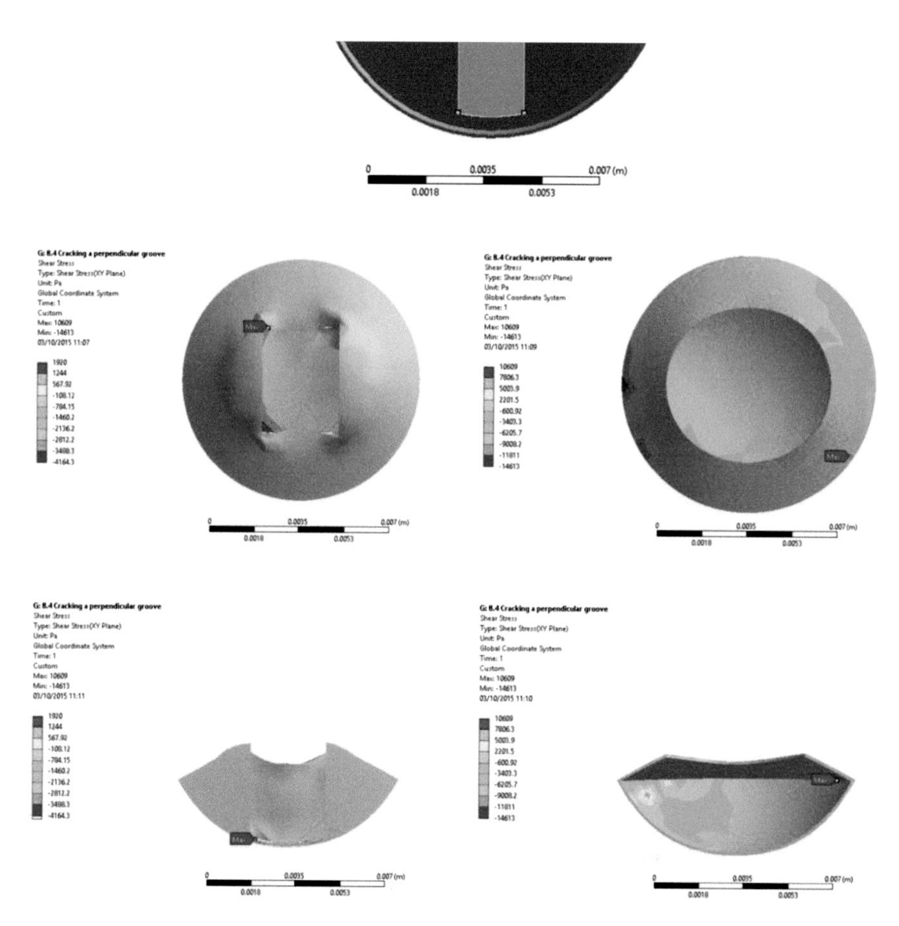

Fig. 4.67 FEA when force is applied at right angles to the side walls of a groove that is sculpted perpendicular to the lens plane, and when the lens plane is at neutral position, in such circumstances the shear stress generated at the nucleus is 0.18 of that generated in the capsule. *Top* shows the position of the lens in relation to the applied force. *Middle left* shows the level of shear stress in the lens (*top view*). *Middle right* shows the level of shear stress in the capsule (*top view*). *Bottom left* shows the level of shear stress (*side view*). *Bottom right* shows the level of shear stress in the capsule (*side view*)

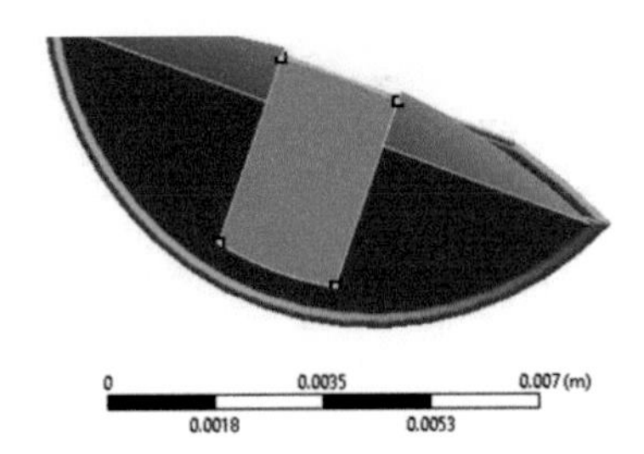

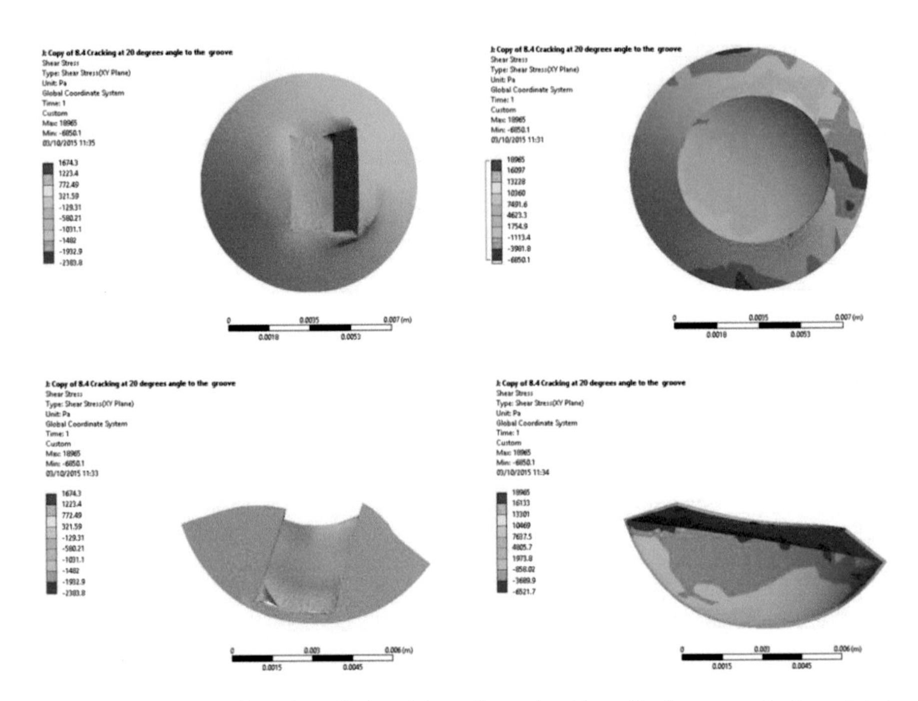

Fig. 4.68 FEA when force is applied at right angles to the side walls of a groove that is sculpted perpendicular to the lens plane, but the lens plane is tilted by 20°, in such circumstances the shear stress generated at the nucleus is 0.01 of that generated in the capsule. *Top* shows the position of the lens in relation to the applied force. *Middle left* shows the level of shear stress in the lens (*top view*). *Middle right* shows the level of shear stress in the capsule (*top view*). *Bottom left* shows the level of shear stress (*side view*). *Bottom right* shows the level of shear stress in the capsule (*side view*)

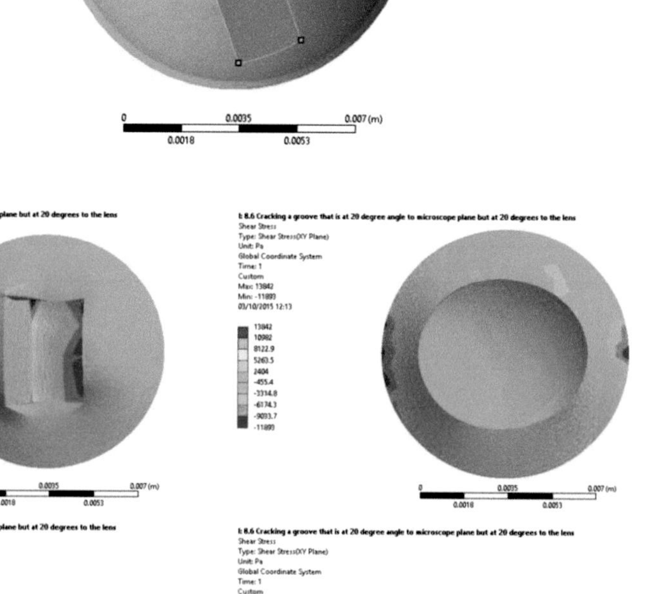

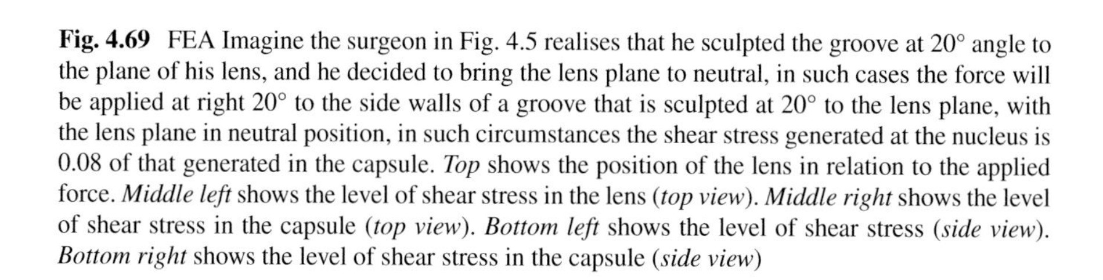

Fig. 4.69 FEA Imagine the surgeon in Fig. 4.5 realises that he sculpted the groove at 20° angle to the plane of his lens, and he decided to bring the lens plane to neutral, in such cases the force will be applied at right 20° to the side walls of a groove that is sculpted at 20° to the lens plane, with the lens plane in neutral position, in such circumstances the shear stress generated at the nucleus is 0.08 of that generated in the capsule. *Top* shows the position of the lens in relation to the applied force. *Middle left* shows the level of shear stress in the lens (*top view*). *Middle right* shows the level of shear stress in the capsule (*top view*). *Bottom left* shows the level of shear stress (*side view*). *Bottom right* shows the level of shear stress in the capsule (*side view*)

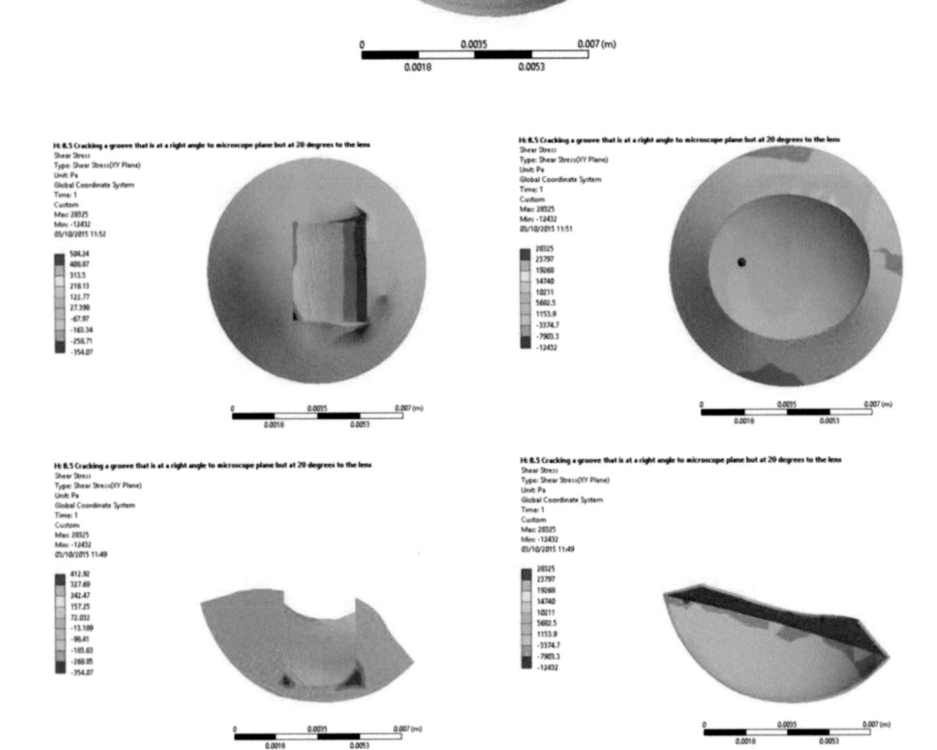

Fig. 4.70 FEA When force is applied at right angles to the side walls of a groove that is sculpted at 20° to the lens plane, and the lens plane kept tilted by 20°, in such circumstances the shear stress generated at the nucleus is 0.02 of that generated in the capsule. *Top* shows the position of the lens in relation to the applied force. *Middle left* shows the level of shear stress in the lens (*top view*). *Middle right* shows the level of shear stress in the capsule (*top view*). *Bottom left* shows the level of shear stress (*side view*). *Bottom right* shows the level of shear stress in the capsule (*side view*)

References

1. Hermans E, et al. Change in the accommodative force on the lens of the human eye with age. Vision Res. 2008;48(1):119–26.
2. Gimbel HV, Neuhann T. Development, advantages, and methods of the continuous circular capsulorhexis technique. J Cataract Refract Surg. 1990;16(1):31–7.

Chapter 5
Compartments

When considering the eye for surgical purposes it is useful to divide the eye into surgical compartments, for example a membrane made up of the lens zonules, the lens and the lens capsule effectively divides the eye into an anterior and posterior compartments. This compartmentalization affects how to the eye will respond during operations. A common situation is an anterior wound and surgical manipulation in the anterior segment. Insertion of fluid into the anterior chamber causes egress of fluid from the wound or posterior movement of the lens diaphragm. If the flow of fluid is balanced inflow and outflow, the posterior segment remains unaffected and stable. Indentation of the wall of the anterior chamber is compensated by flow of fluid out of the wound and the posterior segment is unaffected. In contrast, pressure on the posterior segment by indentation may cause movement of the membrane towards the anterior segment, if a wound exists in the anterior segment, and then both compartments are affected (Figs. 5.1, 5.2, 5.3, 5.4 and 5.5).

FEA Pressure Balance on Both Sides

Once the corneal section is performed the balance between the front and the back surface of the lens starts to change. Injecting viscoelastic material in to the anterior chamber helps to neutralise this balance. Lower pressures in the anterior chamber results in anterior capsular tear extensions while higher pressures in the anterior segments results in posterior capsular extensions (Fig. 5.6).

The eye in order to maintain its shape as a spheroid is required to exist at a pressure higher than the atmospheric pressure (10–21 mmHg). Therefore surgery on the eye often requires the employment of infusion fluids to maintain the pressure. The effects of any infusion cannula will vary depending upon which compartment the infusion is inserted into. Care must be taken that the infusion does not switch between compartments, as the effects of the infusion will be changed. The external

T.H. Williamson, *Intraocular Surgery: A Basic Surgical Guide*,
DOI 10.1007/978-3-319-27990-9_5

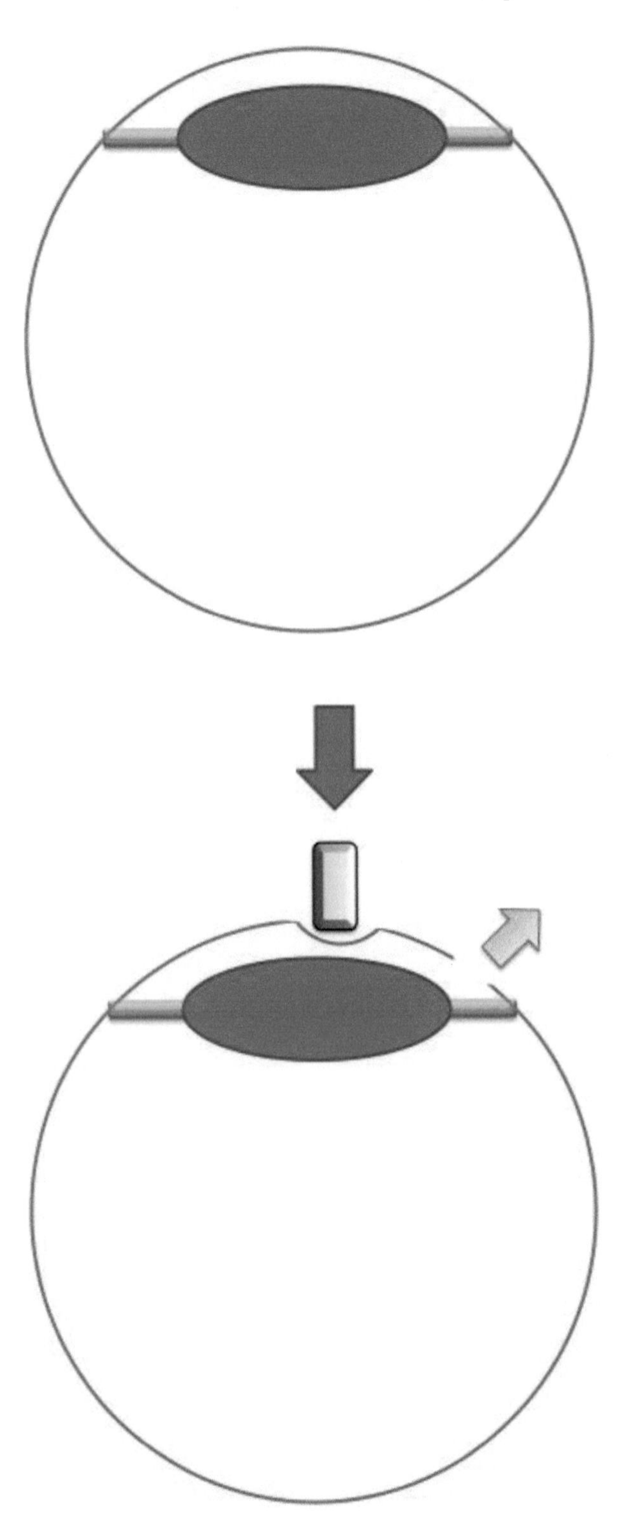

Fig. 5.1 The eye can be considered as two compartments separated by a diaphragm consisting of the lens and its zonules

Fig. 5.2 Pressure on the compartment in which there is a wound affects only that compartment and the other is stable

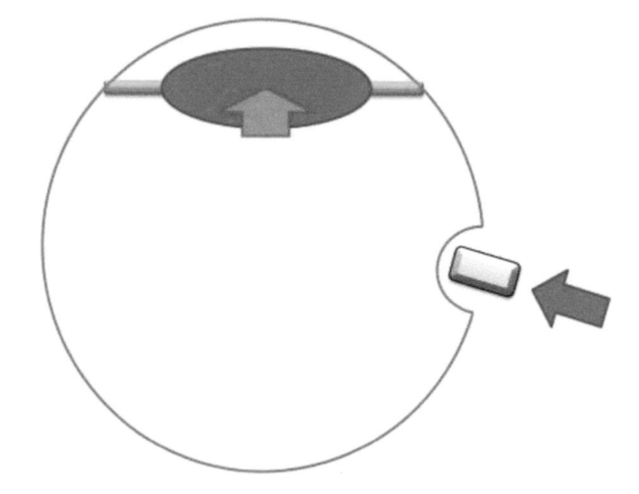

Fig. 5.3 Pressure on the other compartment to the one with the wound can affect both compartments, see below

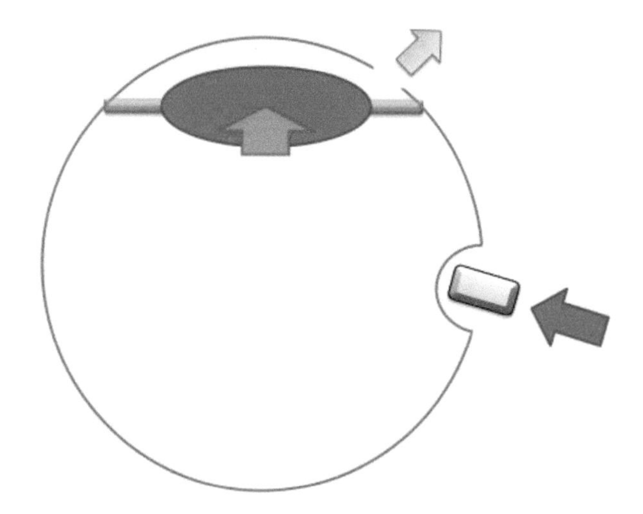

Fig. 5.4 See Fig. 5.3

tubing attached to an infusion can alter the angulation of the infusion. Therefore simply by angling the eye for examination the infusion may be inadvertently relocated into a different compartment, potentially displacing the membrane divides the two compartments. Disorders of the eye such as retinal detachment or choroidal effusion will create yet more compartments, into which an infusion may erroneously be inserted with subsequent consequences for that compartment (Figs. 5.5, 5.6, 5.7, 5.8, 5.9, 5.10, 5.11 and 5.12).

Forces on a compartment will influence a secondary membrane such as a retinal detachment. For example, indentation of the sclera within the elevation of a retinal detachment will have a small effect on movement of the retinal detachment. However if indentation is applied at the junction of the membrane to the wall of the eye and then a much larger movement of the membrane is induced (Figs. 5.13 and 5.14).

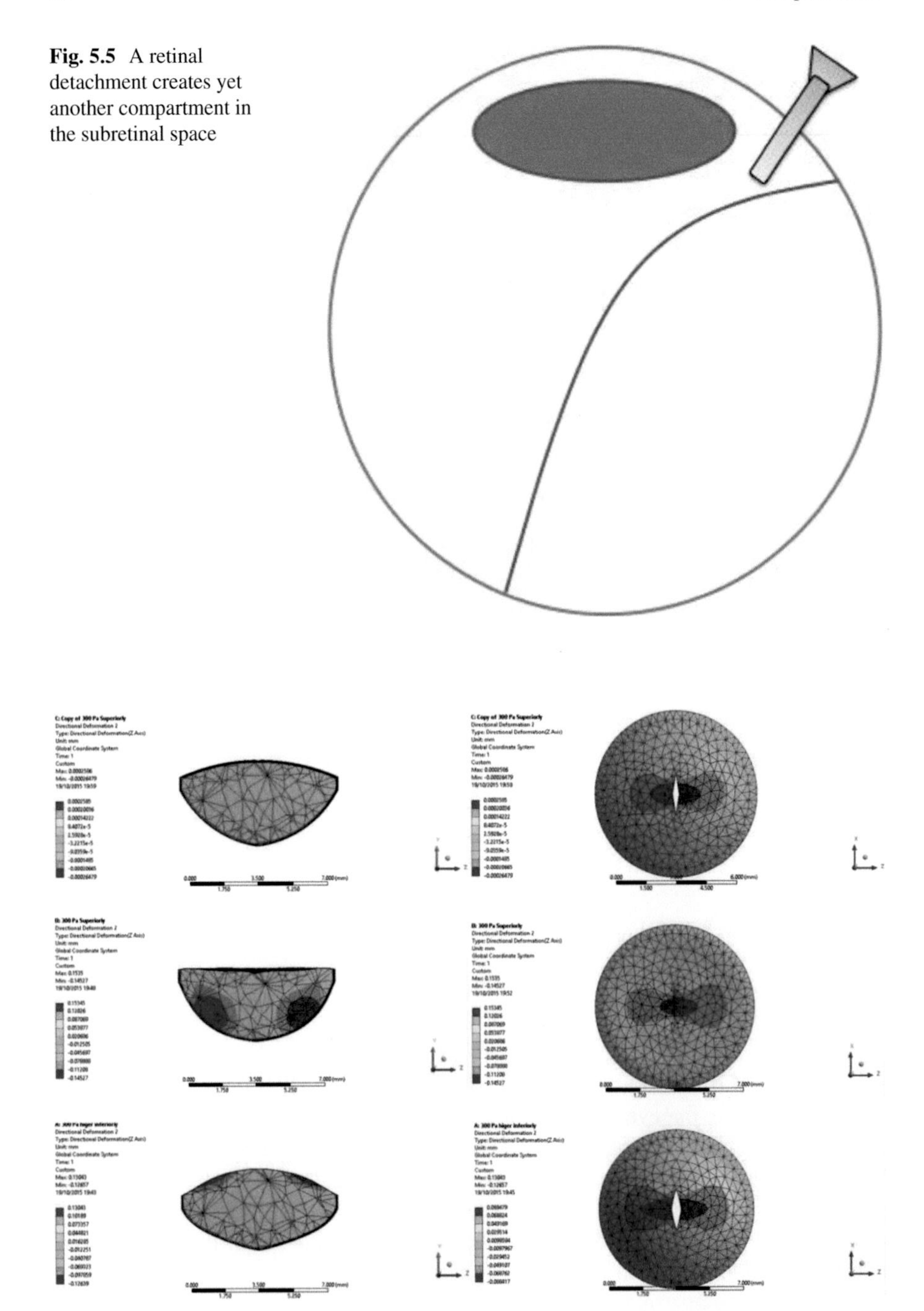

Fig. 5.5 A retinal detachment creates yet another compartment in the subretinal space

Fig. 5.6 When pressure on the nucleus of the lens is neutral the capsules are not put under pressure. High pressure in the anterior chamber puts tension on the posterior capsule (*second row*) and low pressure in the anterior chamber puts tension on the anterior capsule (*third row*)

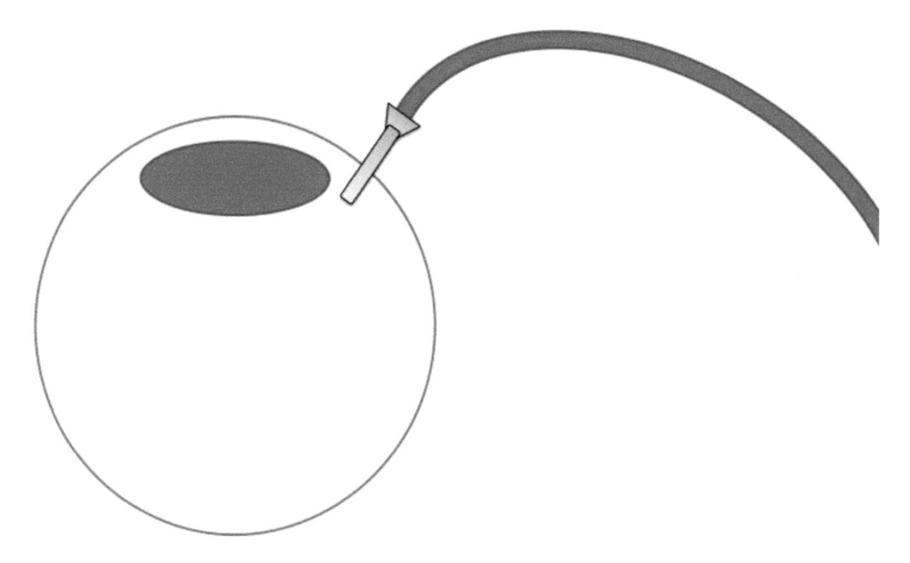

Fig. 5.7 Instruments that have fixed point outside of the eye can rotate and change position on movement of the eye

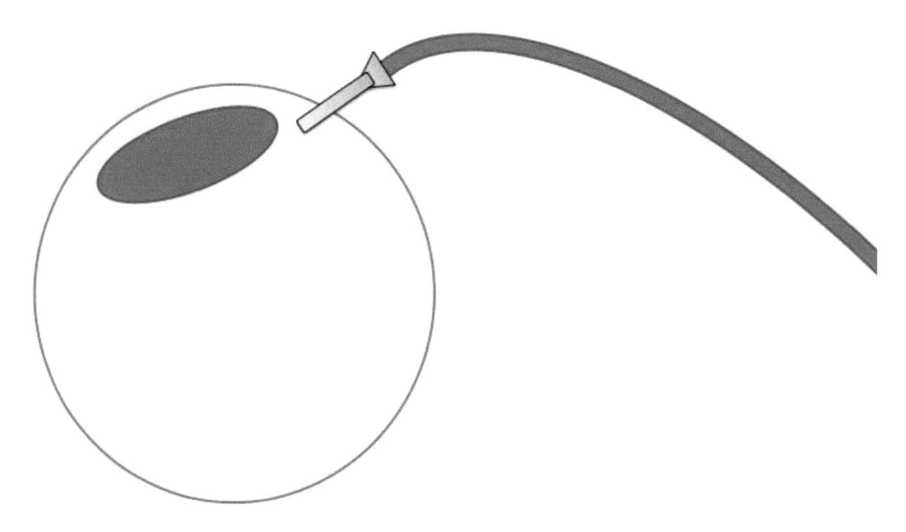

Fig. 5.8 This movement may move the instrument from one compartment to another

Manipulation of one compartment causes pressure rises in that compartment, which are usually compensated for by egress of fluid from a wound or passage of fluid into an infusion port. In order to minimise pressure fluctuations and ingress and egress of fluid, indentations should be kept constant but can be moved around the wall of the globe whilst maintaining the pressure. In other words, it is better to move an instrument whilst maintaining pressure rather that releasing and reapplying pressure excessively (Figs. 5.15 and 5.16).

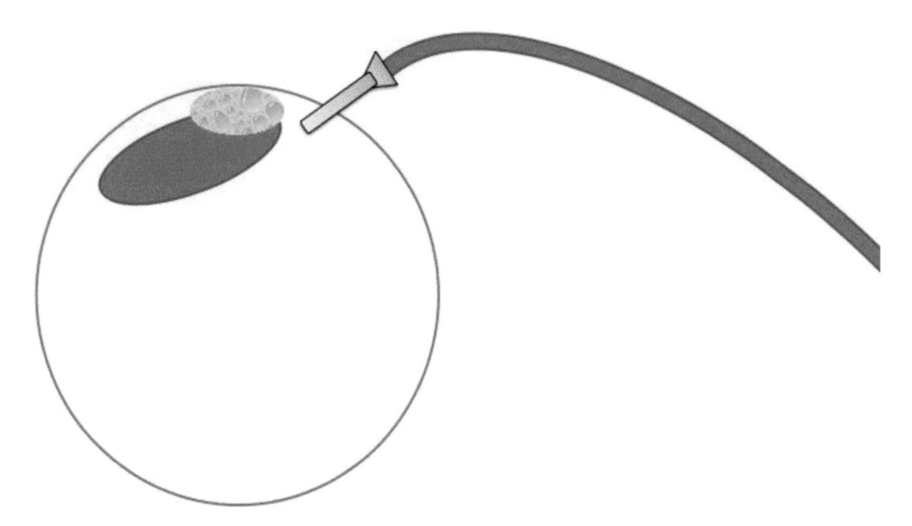

Fig. 5.9 This can involve infusion, e.g. gas, into the wrong compartment

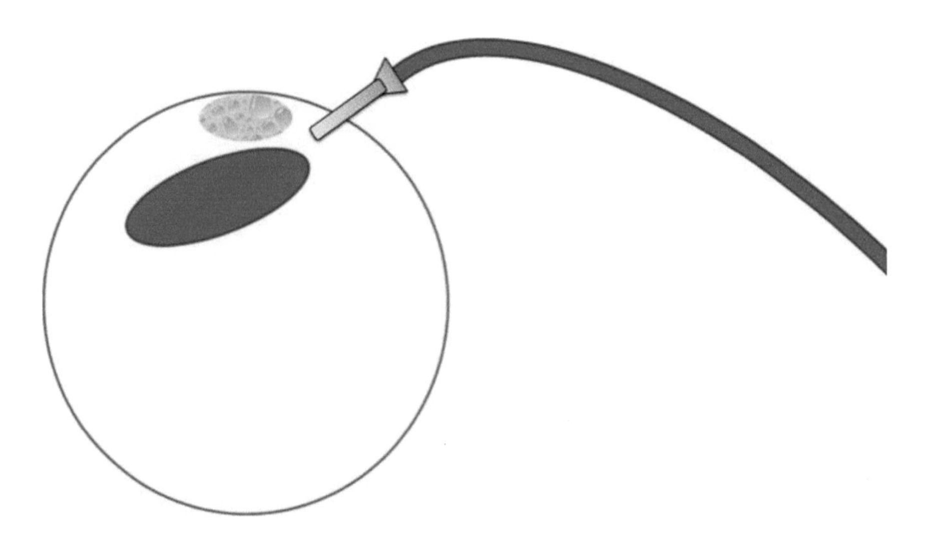

Fig. 5.10 This may distort the compartment membrane

FEA Choroidal Haemorrhage

Choroidal haemorrhage usually occurs usually in the suprachoroidal space is a potentially devastating complication of cataract surgery. The incidence of which is 0.04 % in cataract surgery and 0.17 % of vitreoretinal surgery [1, 2]. Most authors consider ocular hypotony to be essential in the development of Choroidal haemorrhage [3, 4]. The evidence shows that choroidal haemorrhage occurs most frequently after removal of the nucleus in extra-capsular cataract extraction. Hypotony induced during nuclear expression is considered to be the reason [2, 5, 6].

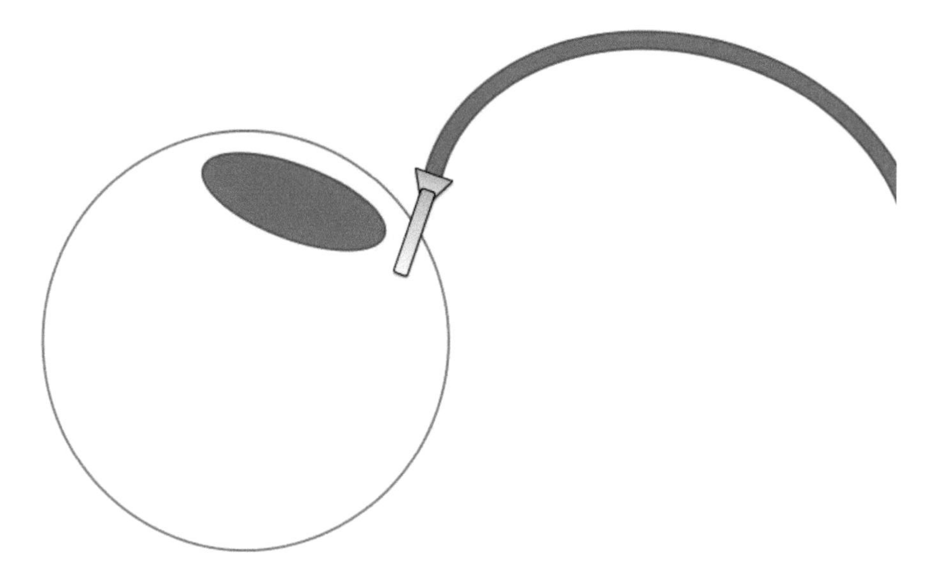

Fig. 5.11 The infusion may move posteriorly

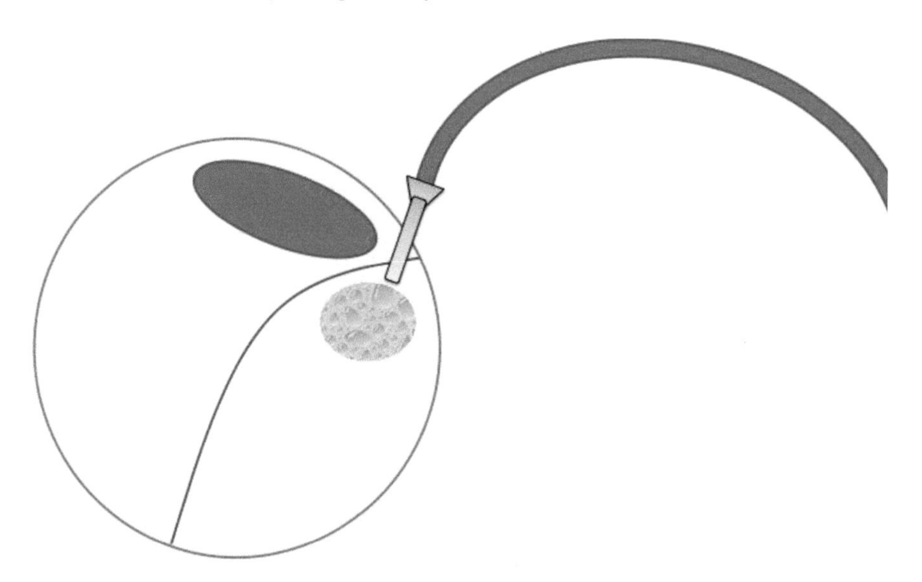

Fig. 5.12 This may cause infusion into the subretinal compartment

However distortion of the globe also plays a role in development of choroidal haemorrhage. Maximal distortion takes place during nuclear expression. Scleral explant application in vitreoretinal surgery also causes globe distortion and is also associated higher risk of choroidal haemorrhage [7–9].

Finite element analysis shows that while 30 % increment in the pressure at arteriolar end of capillary and reducing the intraocular pressure to zero both independently increase the shear stress in the capillary blood vessels by one to two folds, mechanically stretching the capillaries by 4 % will result in 43 fold increase in shear

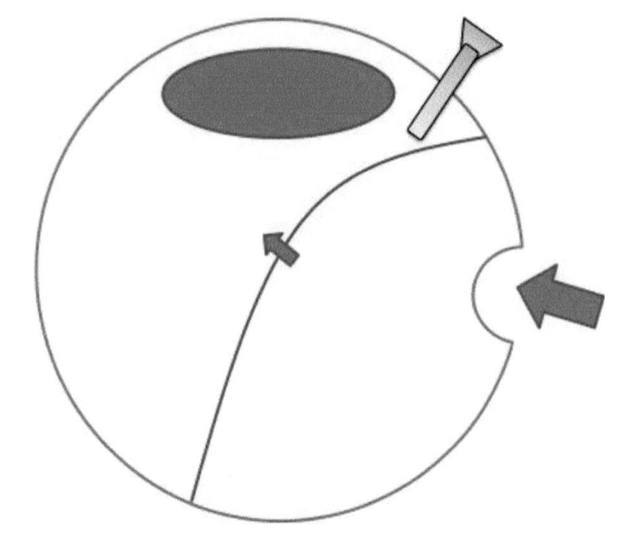

Fig. 5.13 Pressure on a compartment wall which is far away from the insertion of the diaphragm (retina in this case) causes minimal movement of the diaphragm

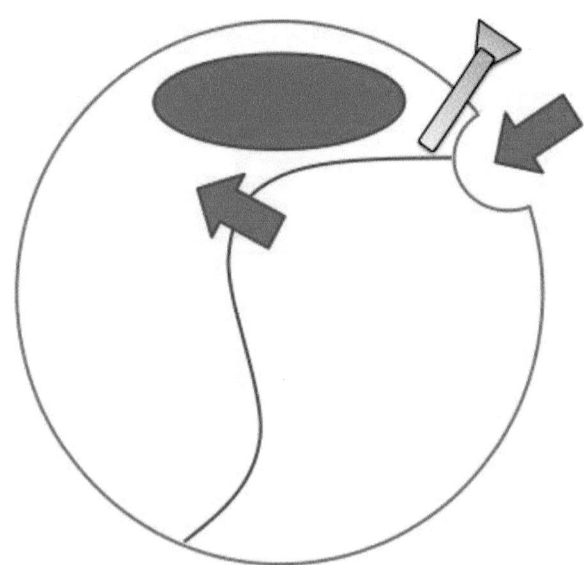

Fig. 5.14 Indentation near the insertion of the diaphragm causes a large movement in the diaphragm risking complications

stress in the capillary wall, this emphasizes the role of globe distortion during surgery in developing choroidal hemorrhage.

It is useful to think about the eye as a fragile tissue that can break or tear if handled carelessly during the operation. Therefore do not distort the globe and take care when indenting and tightening sutures over an external buckle. Think 'I do not want to fracture a blood vessel'. Also it is important to maintain intraocular pressure during the entire length of surgery.

Important considerations when choroidal hemorrhage arises

1. Stop leakage and maintain intraocular pressure.
2. Raise the pressure in the globe.

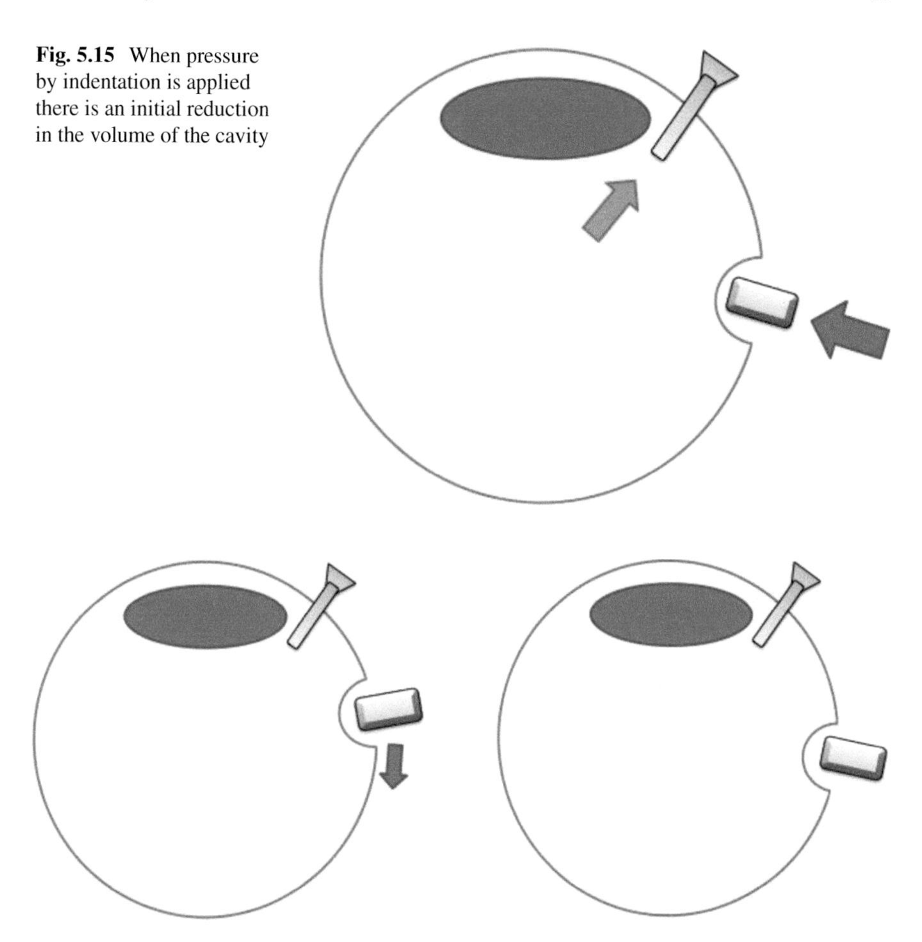

Fig. 5.15 When pressure by indentation is applied there is an initial reduction in the volume of the cavity

Fig. 5.16 By maintaining the pressure whilst moving the indentation no further volumetric changes are required and the cavity is stable

3. Allow time for a clot to form.
4. Finish the operation and close.
5. if a fill of the eye is required liquid is better than gas as the former is non-compressible (Fig. 5.17).

Arc of Safety

Inserting instruments into the internal volume of sphere creates certain dynamics, which should be understood. In most circumstances in intraocular surgery, the instrument is anchored in its movement at its point of insertion into the globe. This influences how the instrument can be moved around within the sphere. The maximum insertion of the instrument is when the instrument passes through the centre of the sphere, and any movement from this position risks impact of the instrument on

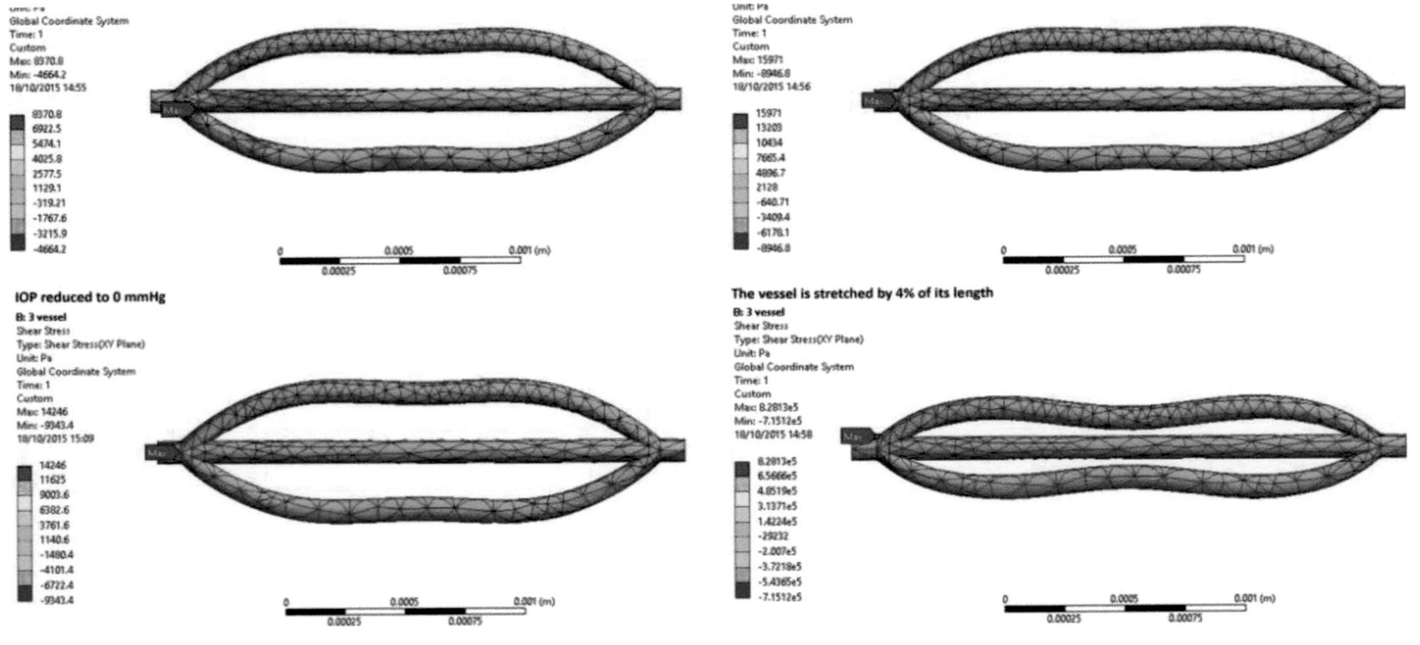

Fig. 5.17 Finite element analysis shows that while a 30 % increase in the pressure at arteriolar end of capillary or reducing the intraocular pressure to zero both independently increase the shear stress in the capillary blood vessels by one to two fold, mechanically stretching the capillaries by 4 % will result 43 fold increase in shear stress in the capillary wall. Upper left shows shear stress at the capillary vessels with intra luminal pressure of 35 mmHg and intra-ocular pressure of 15 mmHg. Upper right shows shear stress at the capillary vessels with intra luminal pressure of 46 mmHg and intra-ocular pressure of 15 mmHg. Lower left shows shear stress at the capillary vessels with intra luminal pressure of 35 mmHg and intra-ocular pressure of zero. Lower right shows shear stress at the capillary vessels with intra luminal pressure of 35 mmHg and intra-ocular pressure of 15 mmHg being stretched by 4 % of its horizontal length

the interior wall of the sphere. The surgeon therefore needs to make a compensating retraction of the instrument. Elongated eyes with long axial length may require more adjustment of the insertion of the instrument when moving anteriorly and less adjustment when moving posteriorly. Small globes will require a more rapid adjustment on the instrument (Figs. 5.18, 5.19, 5.20, 5.21, 5.22, 5.23 and 5.24).

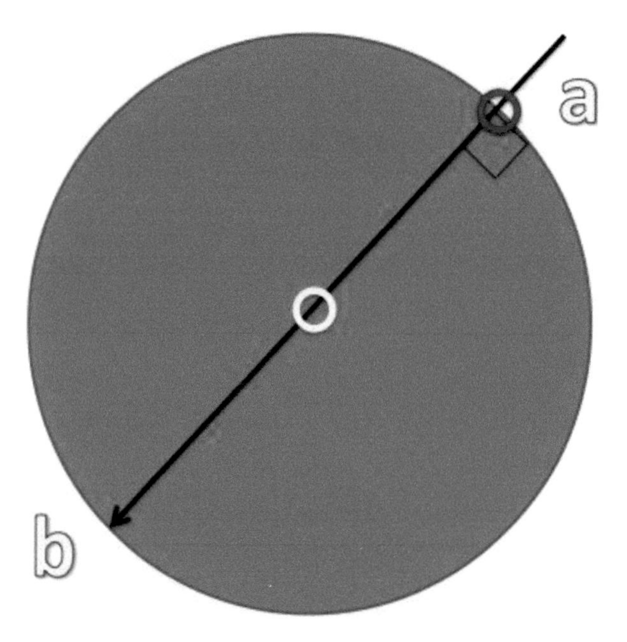

Fig. 5.18 Most instruments in the eye are restricted in their movement by the wound through which they are inserted (*red circle*). The furthest the instrument can be inserted is through the centre of the sphere. If in this position the instrument cannot be moved laterally without touching the wall of the sphere, see below

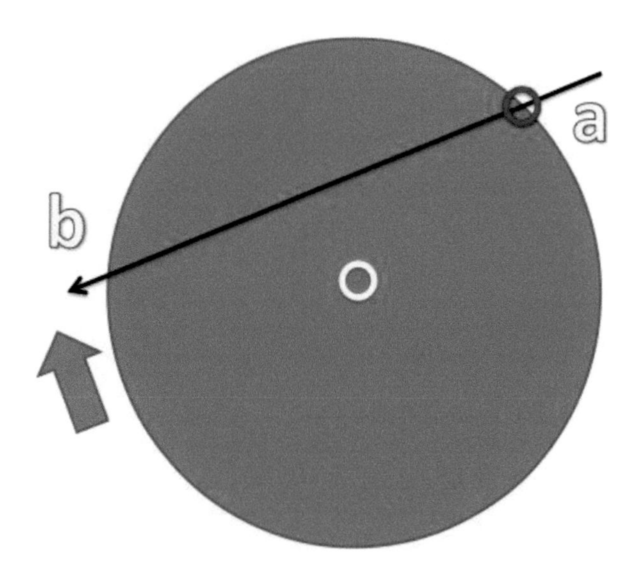

Fig. 5.19 See Fig. 5.18

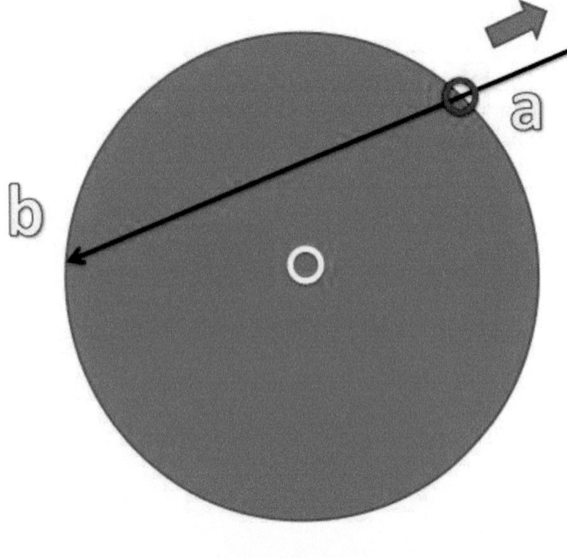

Fig. 5.20 There must be a compensatory retraction of the instrument to allow it to be moved

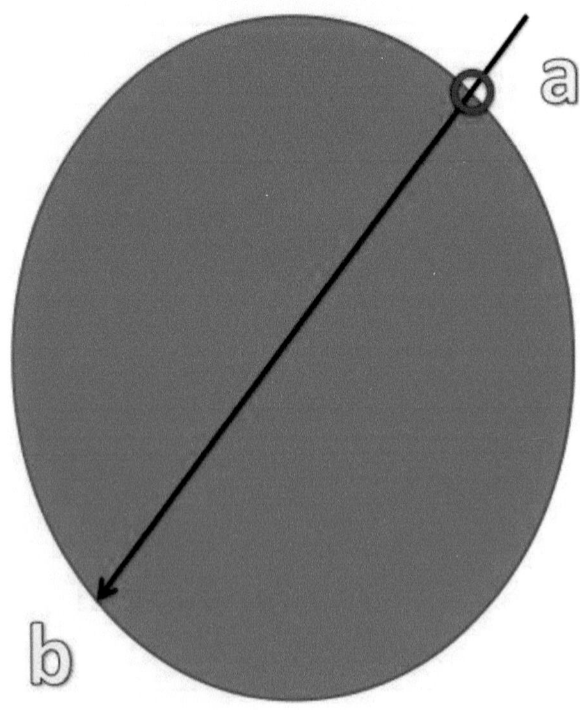

Fig. 5.21 In an oblong eye the safe movement of the instrument is asymmetrical

The instrument rotates around the point of insertion, and therefore an arc of safety can be described centred on the insertion point. When the instrument tip is a certain distance away from the surface of the inside of the globe, movement of the instrument is safe along an arc. In a smaller eye the arc has a smaller radius, in a larger eye it has a larger radius. In an spheroidal eye with elongated axial length the

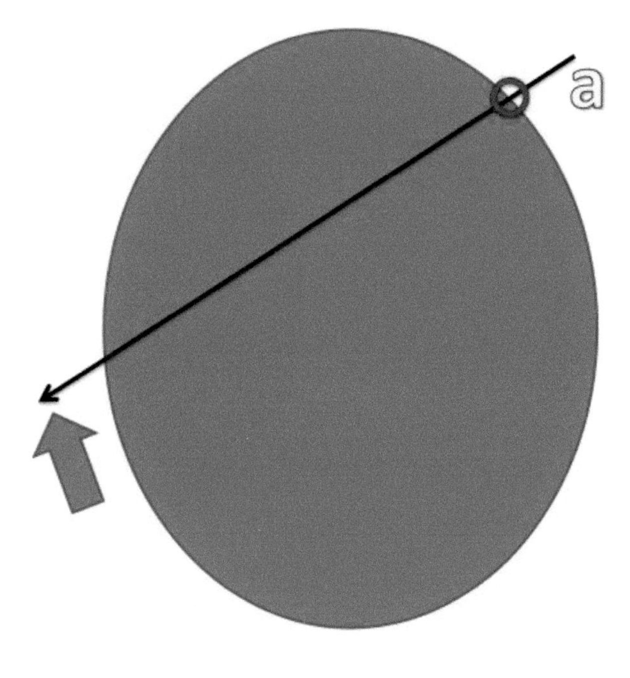

Fig. 5.22 Anterior movement is more restricted

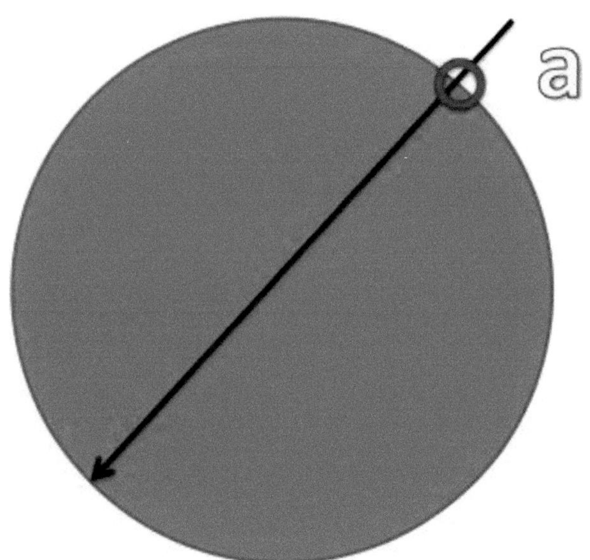

Fig. 5.23 In smaller eyes the movement of the instrument is further restricted, see below

arc of safety demonstrates the asymmetry causing a higher risk of instrument contact going anteriorly than posteriorly (Figs. 5.25, 5.26, 5.27, 5.28, 5.29, 5.30 and 5.31).

For the anterior segment surgeon operating within the lens capsule the arc of safety is very short because of the small size and the shape of the lens. Therefore the cataract surgeon must learn to dynamically manipulate his instrument within this confined area. A J-shaped movement of the instrument is required to operate on the lens whilst avoiding the capsular wall of the cavity (Figs. 5.32, 5.33 and 5.34).

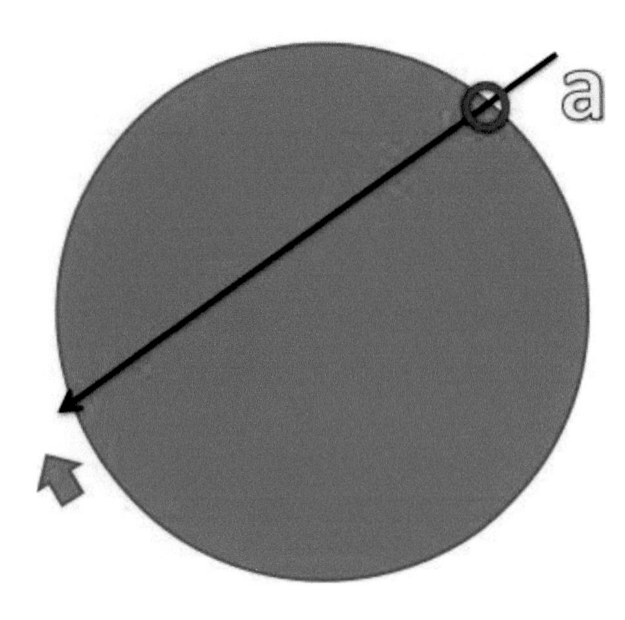

Fig. 5.24 See Fig. 5.23

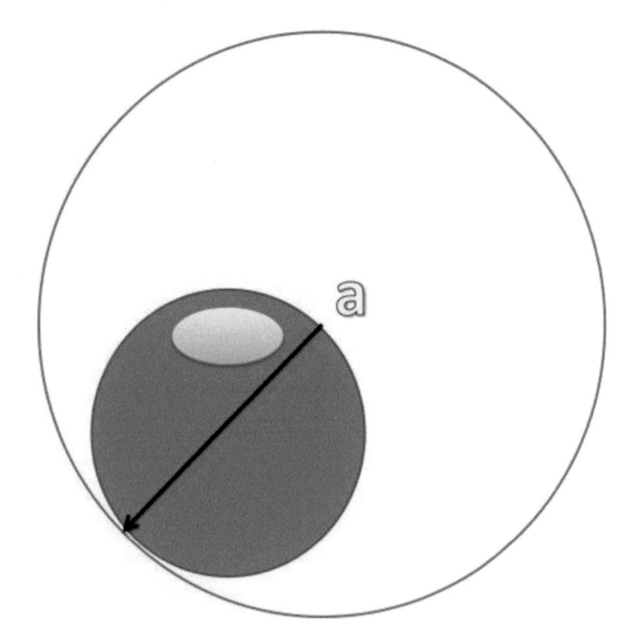

Fig. 5.25 An arc of safety rotating around the wound can be drawn. This arc varies with the size of the eye

FEA Zonular Support

There is a natural tendency to direct the phaco tip deeper as the surgeon comes towards the end of a grooving stroke. This must be resisted because the capsule is least supported just inferior to its periphery (Fig. 5.35).

Fig. 5.26 See Fig. 5.25

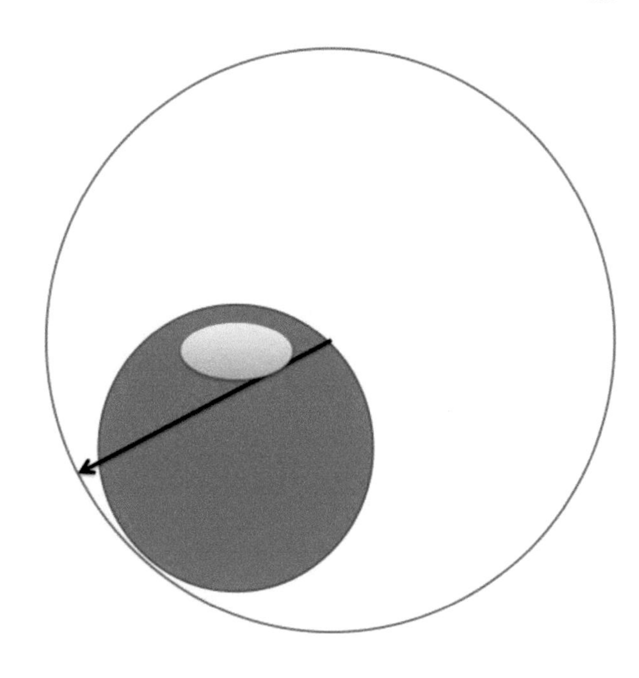

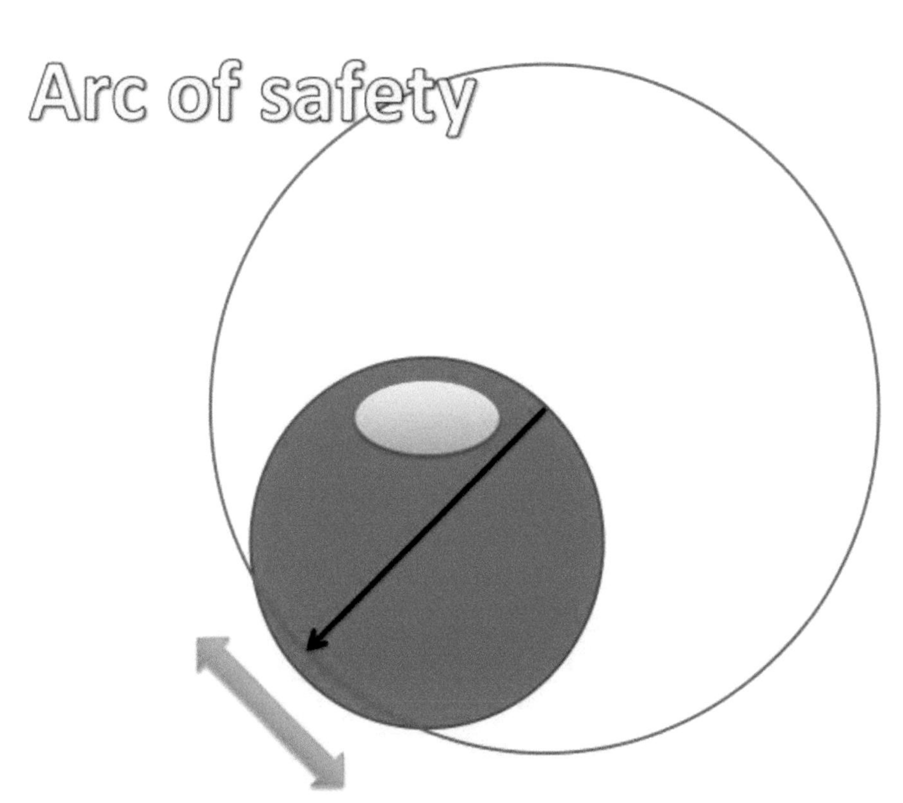

Fig. 5.27 If the arc is kept within the sphere of the eye, there is safe range of movement for the instrument

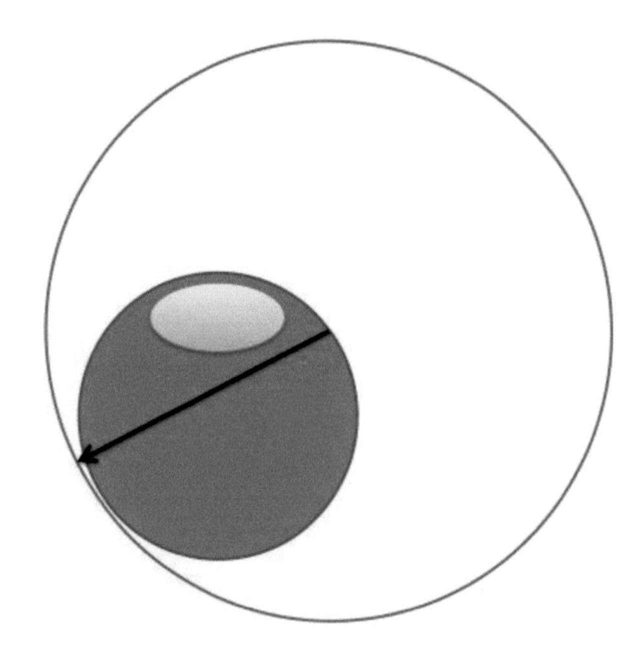

Fig. 5.28 In a smaller eye the instrument will need to be retracted further to achieve the same range of safe usage, see below. The arc of safety has a reduced radius

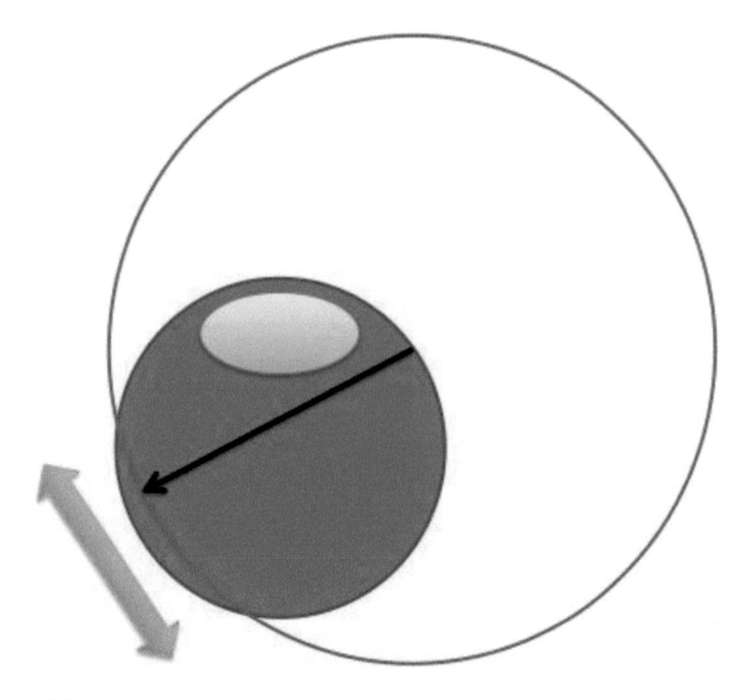

Fig. 5.29 See Fig. 5.28

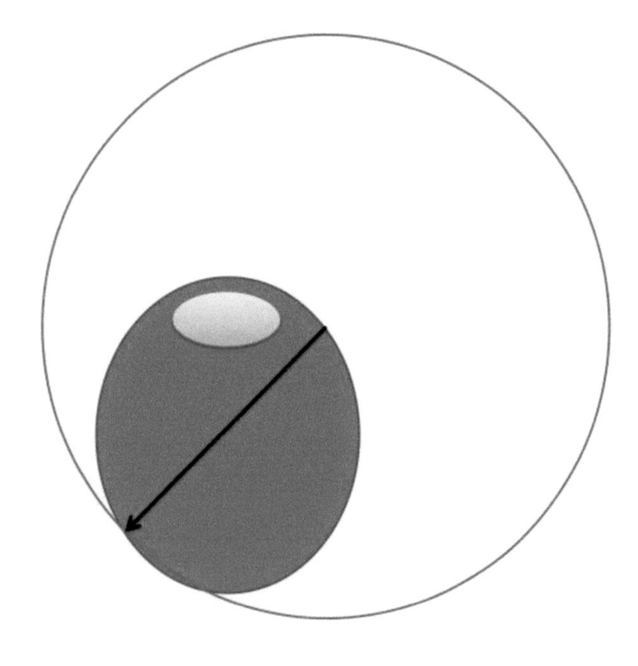

Fig. 5.30 Large oblong eyes will have a larger radius of arc of safety but the arc is more posteriorly placed in the eye, see below

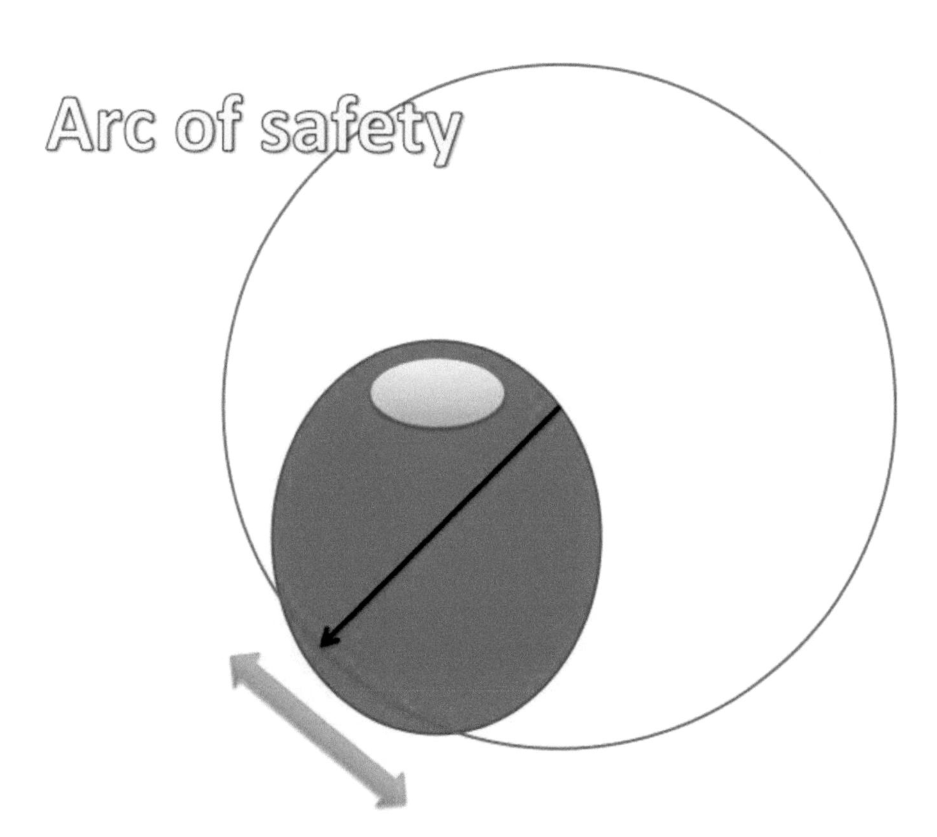

Fig. 5.31 See Fig. 5.30

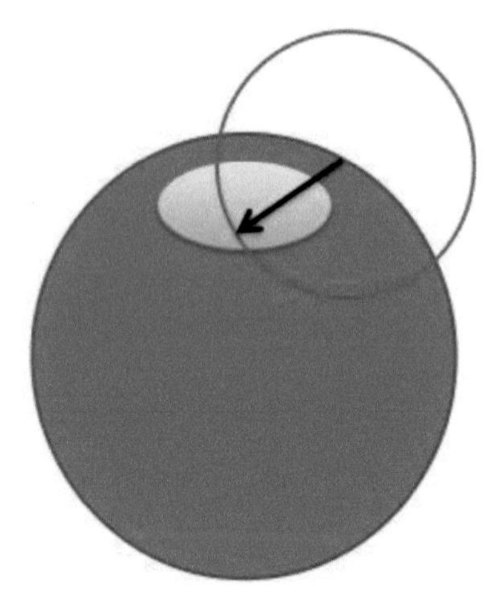

Fig. 5.32 In some compartments such as within the lens capsule the arc of safety is so small the surgeon is obliged to dynamically move the instrument to compensate, see below

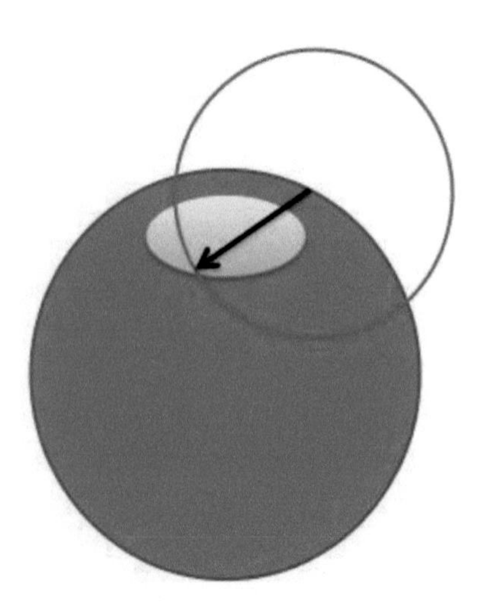

Fig. 5.33 See Fig. 5.32

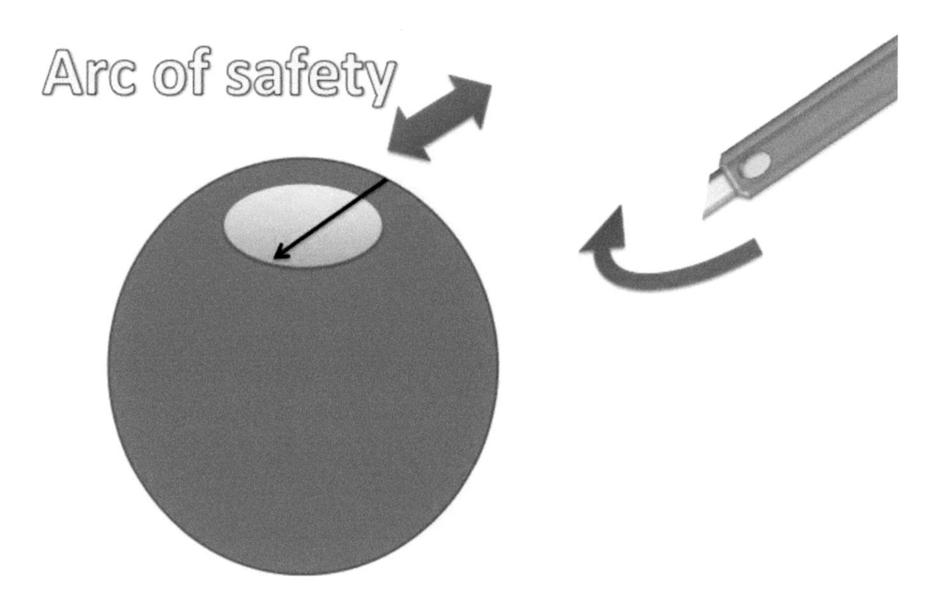

Fig. 5.34 A J-shaped motion is required

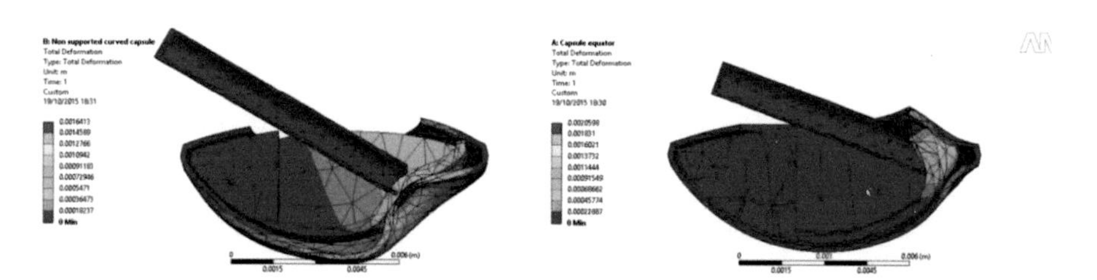

Fig. 5.35 The capsule is least supported at just behind the equator due to its geometry and zonular support and therefore this area should be avoided during aspiration procedures in the anterior chamber

Obstructions in the compartment can affect the arc, for example an instrument in the vitreous cavity anteriorly placed behind the lens has a small arc of safety because the posterior curvature of the lens protrudes into the compartment. The arc is small adjacent to the lens and disappears when the instrument is extended beyond the lens border, but a larger arc of safety is available near the wound itself (Figs. 5.36, 5.37, 5.38, 5.39 and 5.40).

Using two wounds allows the surgeon to overlap arcs of safety. This can help visualisation of the instrument tip and reduce distortion of tissues whilst the surgeon tries to access a particular space. However it carries the disadvantage of creation of extra wounds (Figs. 5.41, 5.42 and 5.43).

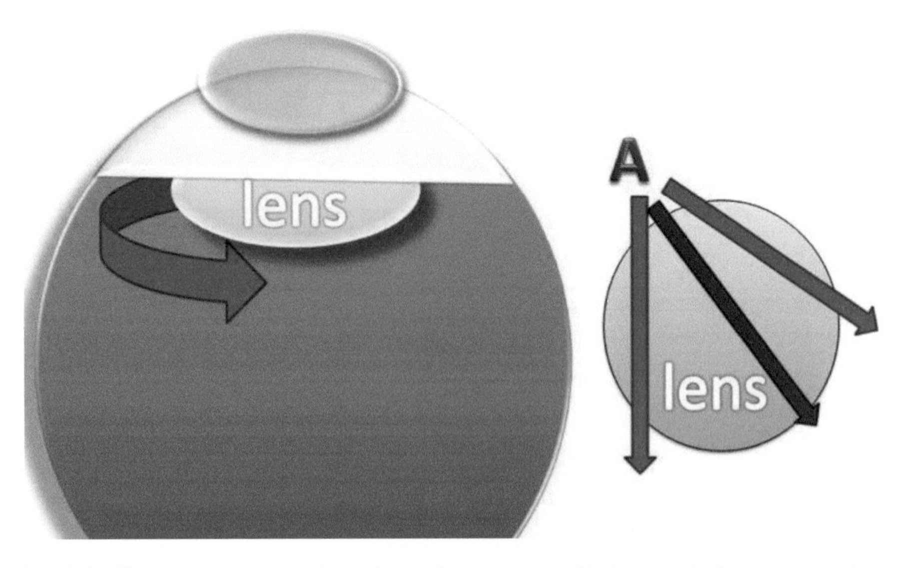

Fig. 5.36 The lens can act as an obstruction to the movement of instruments in the anterior portion of the vitreous cavity (Reprinted from Williamson [7])

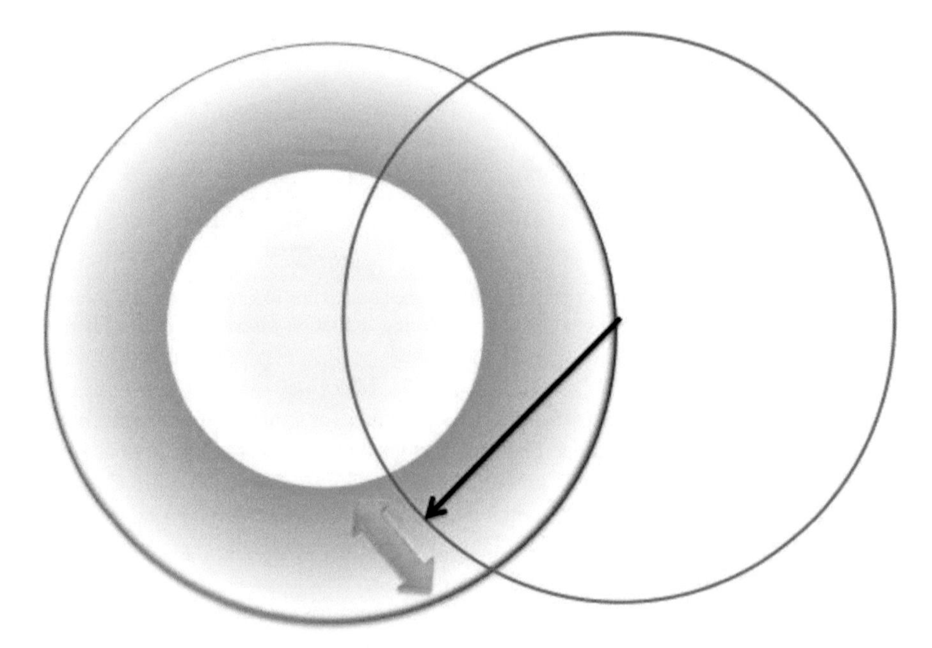

Fig. 5.37 Sometimes a compartment is restricted by another object e.g. the lens in the anterior vitreous cavity. The arc of safety is influenced by the extra object and will vary

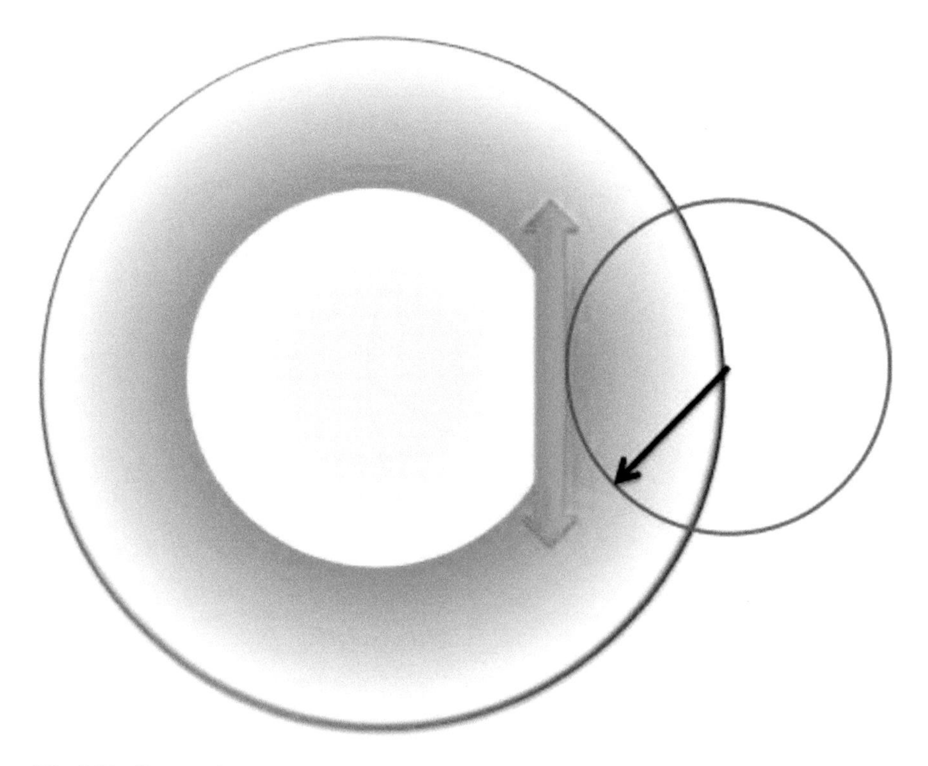

Fig. 5.38 Close to the wound the arc is largest

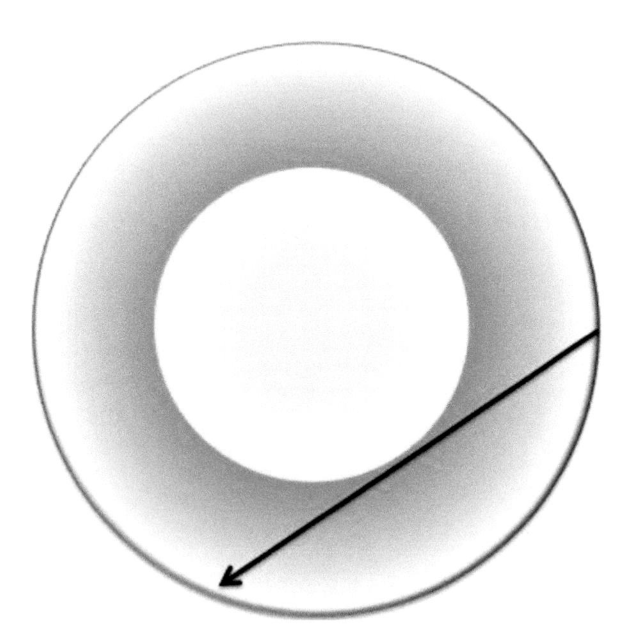

Fig. 5.39 Reaching past the object (e.g. posterior lens) severely restricts mobility, see below

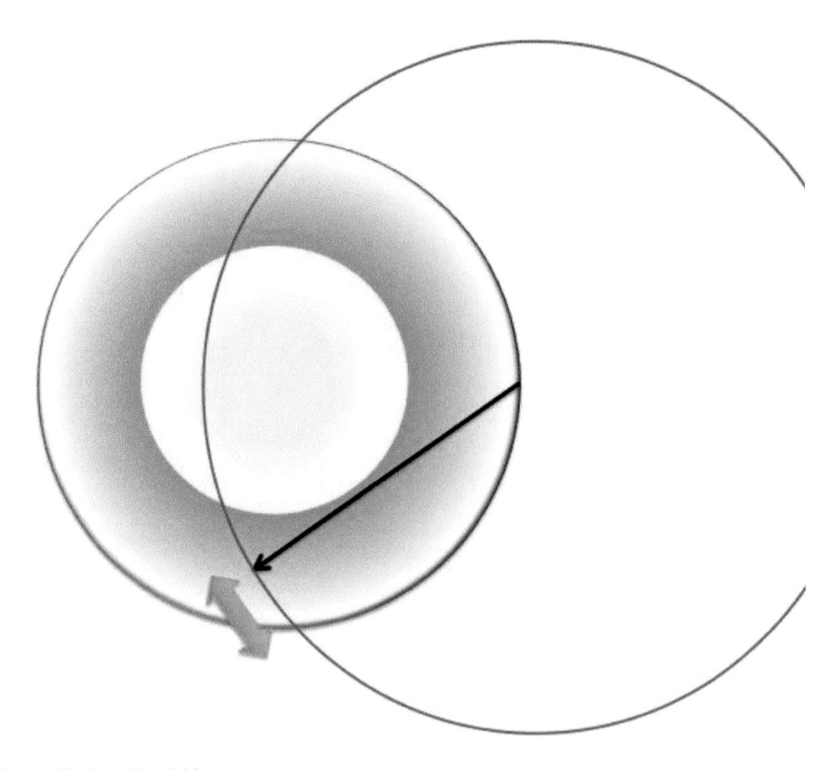

Fig. 5.40 See Fig. 5.39

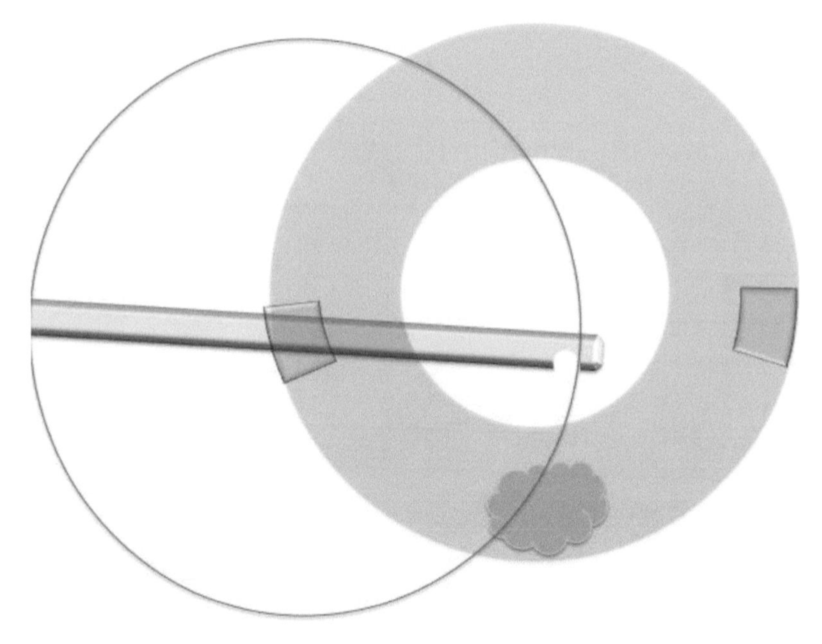

Fig. 5.41 Altering the pivot point (adding a another entry wound) allows a different arc for safe use of the instrument, see below

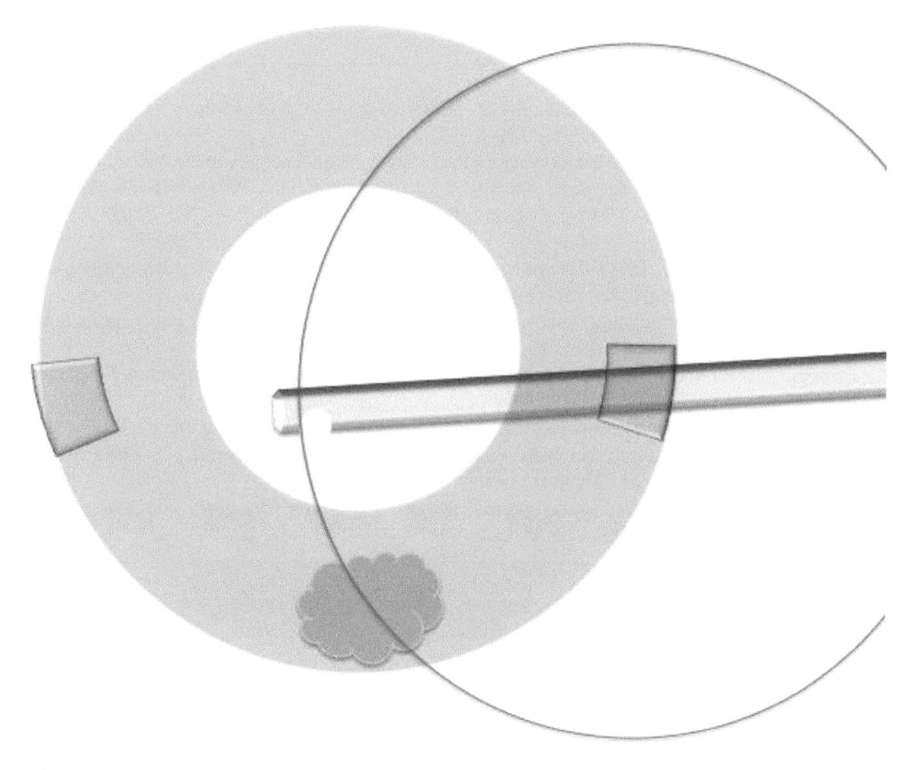

Fig. 5.42 See Fig. 5.41

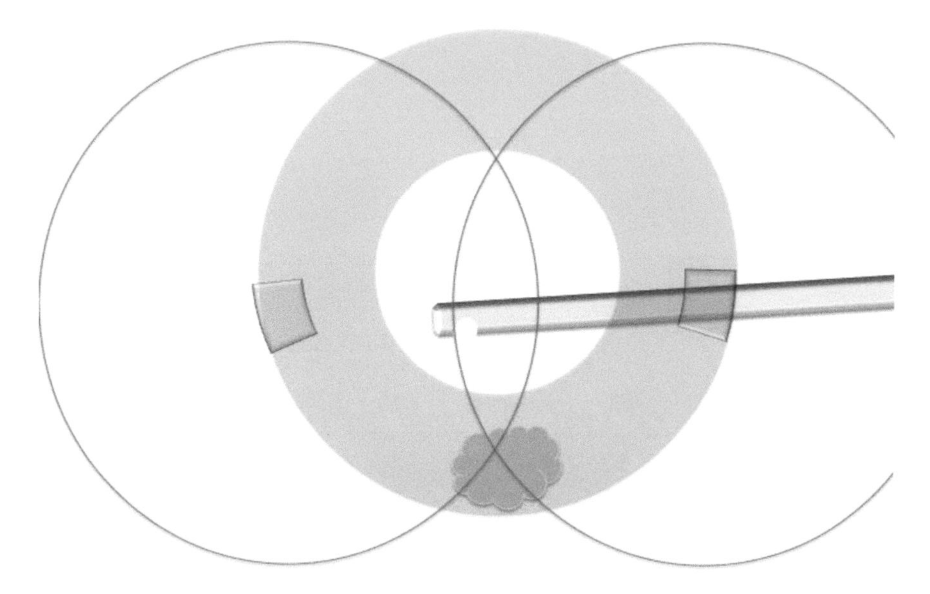

Fig. 5.43 This allow easier access to the whole compartment

References

1. Ghoraba HH, Zayed AI. Suprachoroidal hemorrhage as a complication of vitrectomy. Ophthalmic Surg Lasers. 2000;32(4):281–8.
2. Ling R, et al. Suprachoroidal haemorrhage complicating cataract surgery in the UK: epidemiology, clinical features, management, and outcomes. Br J Ophthalmol. 2004;88(4):478–80.
3. Zauberman H. Expulsive choroidal haemorrhage: an experimental study. Br J Ophthalmol. 1982;66(1):43–5.
4. Beyer CF, Peyman GA, Hill JM. Expulsive choroidal hemorrhage in rabbits: a histopathologic study. Arch Ophthalmol. 1989;107(11):1648–53.
5. Davison JA. Acute intraoperative suprachoroidal hemorrhage in capsular bag phacoemulsification. J Cataract Refract Surg. 1993;19(4):534–7.
6. Eriksson A, et al. Risk of acute suprachoroidal hemorrhage with phacoemulsification. J Cataract Refract Surg. 1998;24(6):793–800.
7. Williamson TH. Vitreoretinal surgery. Berlin: Springer Science & Business Media; 2013.
8. Lakhanpal V, et al. Intraoperative massive suprachoroidal hemorrhage during pars plana vitrectomy. Ophthalmology. 1990;97(9):1114–9.
9. Tabandeh H, Flynn Jr HW. Suprachoroidal hemorrhage during pars plana vitrectomy. Curr Opin Ophthalmol. 2001;12(3):179–85.

Chapter 6
Machines

Complex machinery is used in ophthalmic surgery. The commonest machines in use are for phaco-emulsification and pars plana vitrectomy. They consist of a computer, pumps and instrument devices in the body of the machine and foot pedals to control the functions. In the case of phaco-emulsification the devices include an ultrasonic transducer, and piezo electric crystals that turn electronic signals into mechanical energy. In vitrectomy the devices include guillotine cutters driven by electronic motors or by compressed gas (Fig. 6.1).

In most circumstances the machinery is connected to the eye by tubing. This creates two compartments connected to each other, i.e., the eye and the machine. The utilisation of machinery creates the need to understand flow of fluid in the tubes and pumps. A major function of the machinery is to provide a constant pressure in the globe to maintain safety of the intraocular structures particularly the vascular network. Sudden drops in intra-ocular pressure risk rupture of blood vessel walls and resultant haemorrhage. The eye is connected to the machinery by tubing, which provides a flow of fluid into the eye. The tubing provides a resistance to flow according to the Hagan Poiseuille law.

Hagan Poiseuille Law

$$\text{Volume Flow Rate}(Q) = \frac{\pi d^4 (Pa - Pb)}{L8n}$$

d = diameter of the tube

Pa–Pb = pressure difference between ends of the tube

L = length of the tube

n = viscosity

T.H. Williamson, *Intraocular Surgery: A Basic Surgical Guide*,
DOI 10.1007/978-3-319-27990-9_6

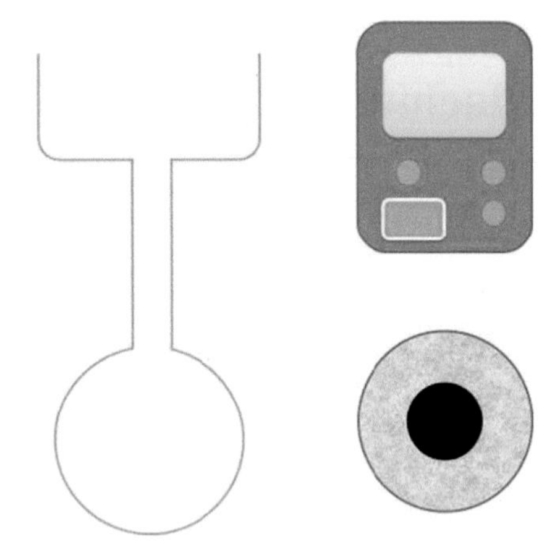

Fig. 6.1 Connecting a piece of machinery to the eye introduces the physics of two compartments joined by a tubing system

Therefore the flow rate is reduced by reduction in the diameter of the tube, by the increased length of the tubing and by increased viscosity of the fluid. The flow is increased by the pressure differential at the ends of the tube, for example,

- Increasing the pressure by raising the height of an infusion bottle relative to the eye or increasing the pump pressure
- Reducing the pressure in the eye by wound leakage or aspiration of fluid.

Another way to envisage the flow of fluid between the compartments is to consider resistance to flow in the system. There is a resistance to inflow from the tubing. There is a resistance to outflow from the eye usually at a wound. Resistance at the wound is reduced when the cross sectional opening of the wound, is largest. A circle provides the largest cross sectional area for a given perimeter therefore a large circular wound has low resistance. Resistance will be reduced by active aspiration of liquid by the action of aspiration pumps. If the resistance to outflow from the globe is greater than the resistance to inflow through the tubing then the pressure in the globe will be maintained. If the resistance at the wound is less than the resistance in the tubing, the pressure in the globe will drop and the structure of the eye collapse (Figs. 6.2 and 6.3).

Flow rate = Velocity × Cross-sectional Area of the tube

In addition manipulations of the globe will affect movement of the fluid between the machine and the eye. For example indentation of the globe will cause a temporary pressure rise until fluid can flow either up the tube or out through the wound. Conversely, release of any indentation will cause a temporary drop in pressure until fluid can be replaced by the inflow. Therefore the rate of change of the globe shape should be performed slowly to allow these adjustments to occur, thereby avoiding sudden changes in pressure. The sphere has the maximal volume for a particular surface area and therefore any deviation from the spherical shape causes a reduction in volume and potential pressure rises (Fig. 6.4).

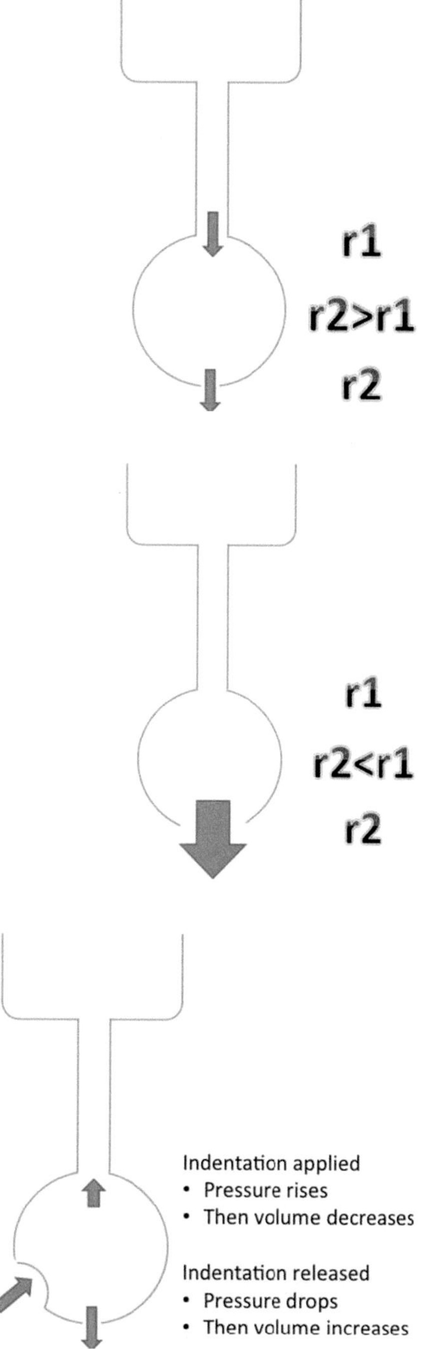

Fig. 6.2 The ocular compartment being a sphere needs to maintain a pressure above atmospheric pressure to maintain its shape. As long as the resistance to inflow of the fluid is less than the resistance to outflow (e.g. a wound) the pressure is maintained

Fig. 6.3 If the resistance to outflow is lower than the resistance to inflow the sphere will collapse

Fig. 6.4 Indentation of the eye increases the pressure before volume is lost up the tubing or out of the wound. Releasing the indentation drops the pressure before the volume is regained from the second compartment via the tubing

Fluids can be allowed to enter the eye passively, for example, by connection to an infusion bottle, in which case the bottle height will relate to the infusion pressure. The height must be measured between the vertical position of the eye and the fluid chamber feeding the infusion line. This can be converted from mmH_2O to mmHg to allow an estimation of the IOP.

Infusion Heights 14 mm $H_2O = 1$ mmHg

Pumps

Alternatively fluids can be allowed to enter by the use of pumps. More commonly however, pumps are used to control fluid egress through instrumentation for example during with the phacoemulsification tip in cataract surgery or the cutter in vitrectomy. Two common types of pumps are utilised. The peristaltic pump involves the production of indentations directly onto the tube enclosing the fluid. These indentions are rotated to move the fluid along the tube. In this type of pump flow is controlled by the rate of rotation of the pump. Increasing the rotations increases the flow of fluid. Vacuum may be created in the tube if the flow is high and there is blockage in the tube preventing flow further down the tubing system. It is important that the tubing cannot collapse as this will lead to a rapid negative pressure on re-expansion of the tube when the blockage is released (Fig. 6.5).

The second type of pump involves flow of a gas along a tubing mechanism. The gas passes along a wide portion of tubing at which point there is a high pressure but low velocity of the gas according to Bernoulli's principal. The introduction of a constriction in the tubing increases the velocity of the gas and consequently the pressure is reduced. At this point the tubing is connected to a compartment and the low pressure created (vacuum) is used to draw fluid into the pump compartment. This type of pump is vacuum controlled and flow is created secondary to the vacuum.

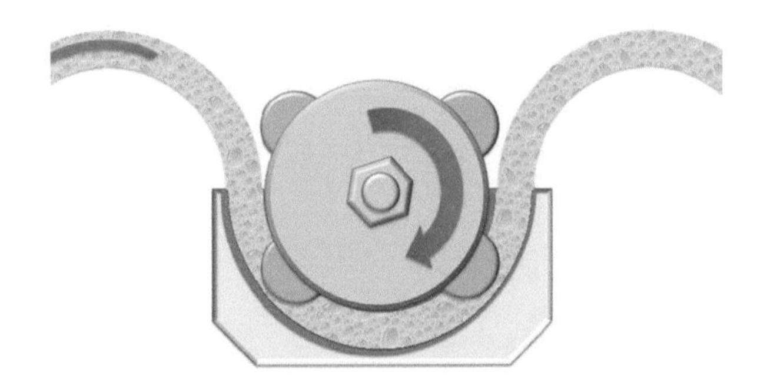

Fig. 6.5 A peristaltic pump creates flow by the action of indentations on the tubing

Bernoulli's Principle states that as the speed of a moving fluid increases, the pressure within the fluid decreases (Fig. 6.6).

$$\text{Pressure} \times \text{velocity} = \text{k}$$

The flow of fluids into the active end of the instrument in the eye creates certain effects. In general, flow is highest in the centre of the tube of an instrument. Liquid at the periphery of the tube is slowed down because of its contact with the wall of the tube. This creates areas of fluid flow around the tip with high velocity (in the centre of the flow) and low velocity (at the periphery). Once again Bernoulli's equation is important because at the border of the tip where the velocity is low the pressure is high, whereas in the centre where the velocity is high the pressure is low. Therefore if the tip is close to a malleable tissue there is the potential for drawing the tissue from the high pressure area to the low pressure area and therefore into the instrument creating injury (Fig. 6.7).

The same principal can be seen at surgical wounds in which there is flow of fluid. The centre of the wound will have high flow and the edge of the wound low flow. The pressure differential created can draw tissue into the wound for example causing iris prolapse into a cataract wound (Fig. 6.8).

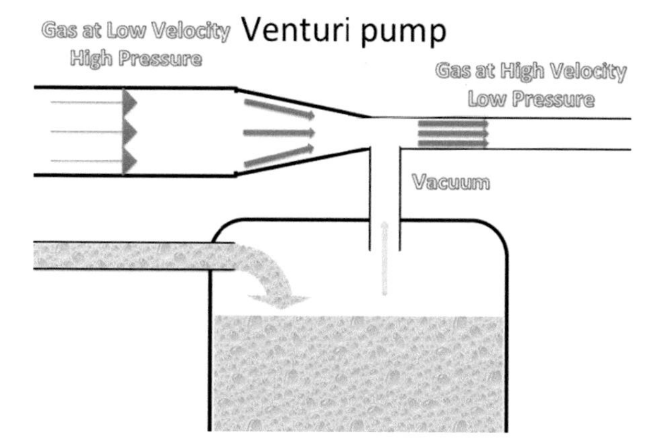

Fig. 6.6 The venturi pump creates a vacuum in a chamber which move the fluid towards the chamber creating flow in the tubing

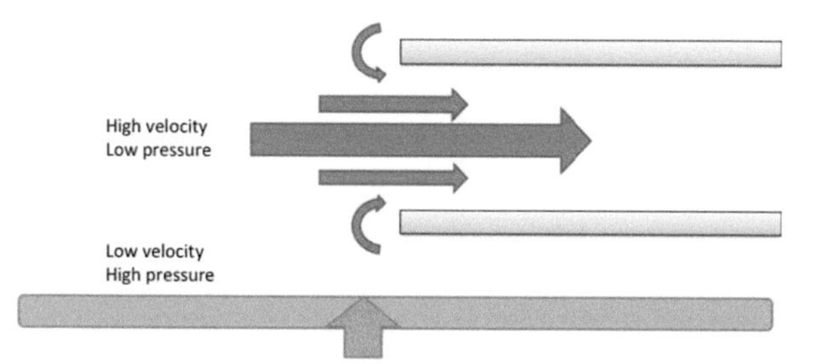

Fig. 6.7 flow of fluid into an aspiration port has higher velocity centrally (*low pressure*) and lower velocity peripherally (*high pressure*). The pressure difference can risk engaging tissue close to the orifice into the port

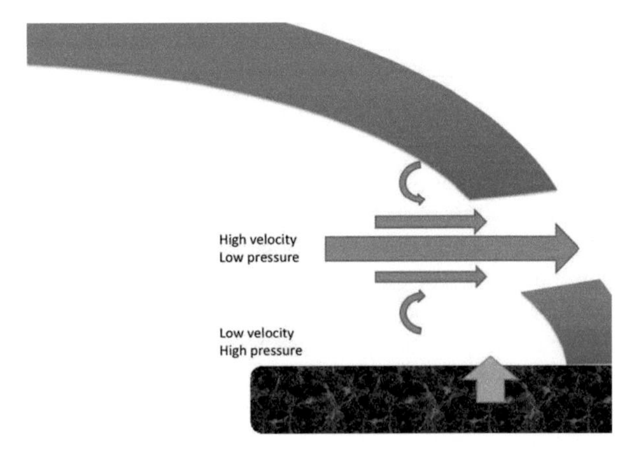

Fig. 6.8 The same effect of flow velocity and pressure can occur at a leaking wound creating lift on a mobile tissue such as the iris leading to prolapse of the tissue

Phacoemulsification

Instrumentation, which is mechanised, is frequently utilised in ocular surgery. The instrumentation is often designed to remove tissue. The tissue characteristics determine how the instrumentation should work. A rapidly oscillating tip, back and forward or side-to-side, can be effective against a hard structure such as the nucleus of the lens. Phacoemulsification tips are made to oscillate at high-frequency (35,000–45,000 Hz) against a hard lens nucleus breaking up the tissue into little pieces (emulsification), which can be aspirated. Two parameters can be altered, the frequency and the stroke length of the movement of the tip. If the frequency is too low the emulsification of the lens is less effective, if the frequency is too high the temperature of the fluid increases. Stroke length is a few thousands of a centimeter and can be varied to increase the emulsification effects.

The phacoemulsification tip acts in two ways to break up the lens nucleus: one by direct impact of the tip on the tissue and the other by the effects of cavitation. The rapid movement of the instrument tip creates cavitation within the fluid, which creates small explosions, which help breakup the hard tissue. As the tip rapidly recedes in the fluid a low-pressure area is created which draws gases out of the liquid creating micro-bubbles. When the tip advances again the tip creates a high pressure which makes most of the bubbles implode releasing energy in the form of shock wave moving in front of the tip, and heat, whilst the remaining micro-bubbles are caught up in the shock wave. Cavitation is related to stroke length with increased stroke length increasing the cavitation effects (Figs. 6.9, 6.10 and 6.11).

Guillotine

The same mechanisms used on a soft tissue such as the vitreous only has the effect of moving the soft tissue away from the tip and therefore does not effectively break down and remove the tissue. Another strategy is required. The vitreous is soft and can be aspirated into a port. Simple aspiration will not work as the tissue has a collagen matrix, which will eventually stop any flow of the tissue in the tubing.

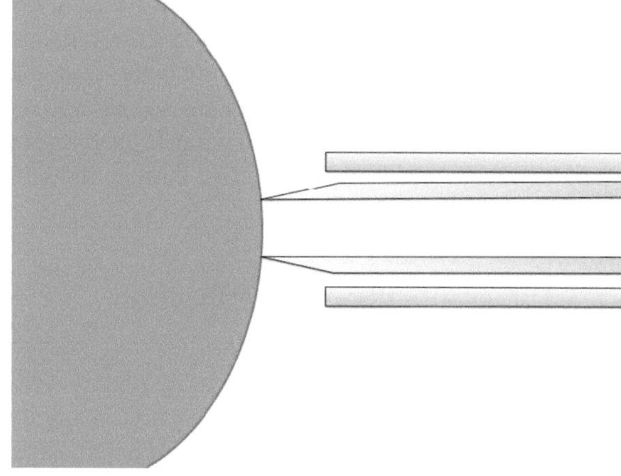

Fig. 6.9 A vibrating blade can be used to break up hard tissue into small pieces (emulsification) to allow its aspiration through a small wound, see below

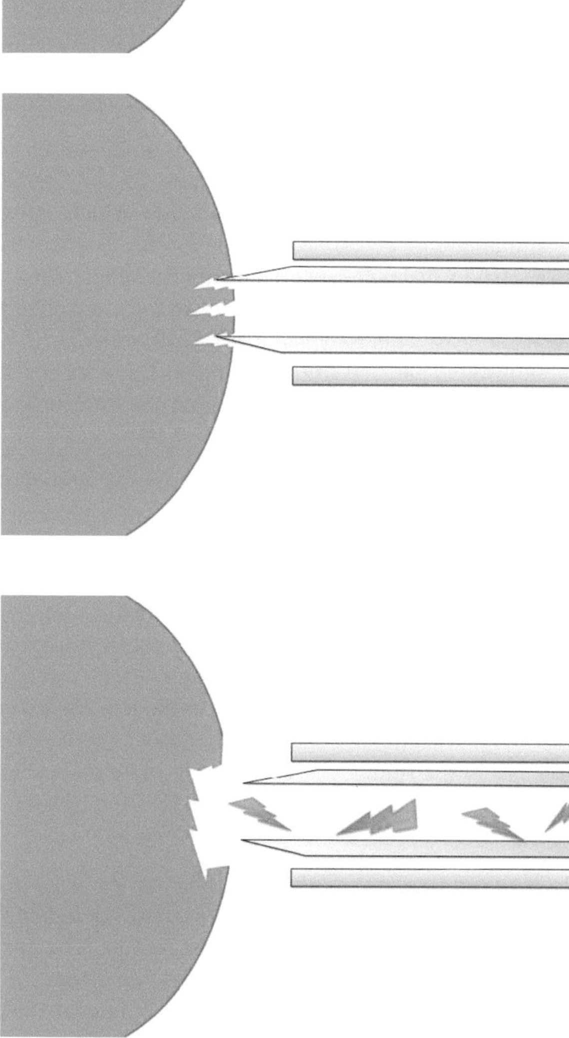

Fig. 6.10 See Fig. 6.9

Fig. 6.11 See Fig. 6.9

Therefore a guillotine cutter slices the soft tissue (cutting the collagen fibrils) into small segments, which are aspirated. Using the same mechanism to remove a hard tissue is ineffective, as the harder tissue cannot be aspirated into the port. This mechanism is often driven forward by compressed gas and returned by the use of springs. The guillotine can only cut the hard tissue if the tissue us presented into the cutter in small fragments, which can be inserted through the orifice of the instrument.

FEA Ultrasonic Phacoemulsification

The phacoemulsification mechanism using high power ultrasound remains the subject of debate. In general tip-tissue interactions occur in "zones" that can be defined moving out from the ultrasonic horn-tip [1]. The zone size depends on ultrasonic horn-tip geometry, the power level and frequency of operations with the distance scale defined by the ultrasound wavelength. The zones are as follows:

1. The tip tissue mechanical interaction zone—which extends less than 500 μm into the impacted tissue.
2. Intermediate mechanical forces zone—which extends in the eye from about a millimetre to a centimetre or more. This is where there are significant radiation pressures that will cause acoustic streaming, debris, or particle motion in fluid.
3. Thermal zone or "far-field"—where the ultrasound is converted to heat through absorption. This is typically, all parts of material beyond those regions where ultrasound interacts in zones 1 and 2. There are also reflections at fluid-tissue and tissue-air interfaces that complicate the ultrasonic field within a limited structure, such as the eye.

Most trainees have no previous experience with ultrasonic cutters. Even if they had previous experience, the performance of a phacoemulsification unit under clinical conditions may not be the same as other ultrasonic cutters used for general purposes. In this section, we are going to simulate the phacoemulsification probe to a hollow tube that heats up when phacoemulsification power is applied. In this simulation the lens and the capsule will behave, as materials that melt and disintegrate when the thermal energy reaches certain levels, just like a candle wax. The capsule however is assumed to be different to the lens by having less thermal conductivity and a higher melting point. The latter assumption is based on the fact that the capsule has lower Young's modulus and is more malleable compared to the lens. This makes it more resistant to phacoemulsification "power" this analogy [2, 3].

The following points would be applicable.

1. No need to apply mechanical force on the lens, if enough phacoemulsfication power is applied and if the probe is close enough to the lens, the lens will start to disintegrate at an area of the initial contact. The initial contact area is usually at the tip of the probe as it is shown in (Fig. 6.16).
2. The disintegrated particles will flow into the phaco probe tip aperture under the influence of the negative pressure generated by the aspiration applied.

3. If the above principle is applied carefully, no movement would be expected in the lens during sculpt ultrasound grooving. If the lens is found to be pushed forward with the action of sculpting this means that the probe is too close to the lens and there is not enough phaco-emulsification power to disintegrate the lens. In such cases the surgeon would need to draw back the probe and applied slightly higher phaco-emulsification power and gradually approach the lens until disintegration in noticed at the leading edge of the phaco-tip. This could be repeated until disintegration is noticed and the particles started to flow into the probe.
4. If the contact between the tip of the probe and the lens is kept to a minimum the risk of posterior capsular rupture would be minimum because the capsule is less likely to be disintegrated by phaco-energy. However, excessive mechanical force applied on the lens during sculpting can risk posterior capsular rupture because the capsule is thinner and more fragile compared to the lens.

Other important considerations in using phacoemulsification

1. There are two types of lateral motion in phacoemulsification

   (a) Torsional motion, in which the phaco tip oscillates in a rotational manner along its primary axis, this type works best with an angled phaco needle.
   (b) Transversal motion, where the phaco tip moves in an elliptical path. This type of motion works equally well with a straight or angled needle.

2. It is important to use as little ultrasonic phaco energy as possible during the cataract surgery. The ultrasonic energy can damage the corneal endothelial cells, with excessive damage leading to corneal decompensation.

The phaco time can be decreased by the following:

(a) Applying the ultrasonic power only when cataract pieces are at the phaco tip and vacuum alone is insufficient to aspirate the piece.
(b) Delivering shorter pulses or bursts of phaco power instead of continuous ultrasound power
(c) Decreasing the duty cycle (the ratio of the on: off pulses) (Figs. 6.12, 6.13, 6.14, 6.15, 6.16, 6.17, 6.18, 6.19, 6.20, 6.21, 6.22 and 6.23)

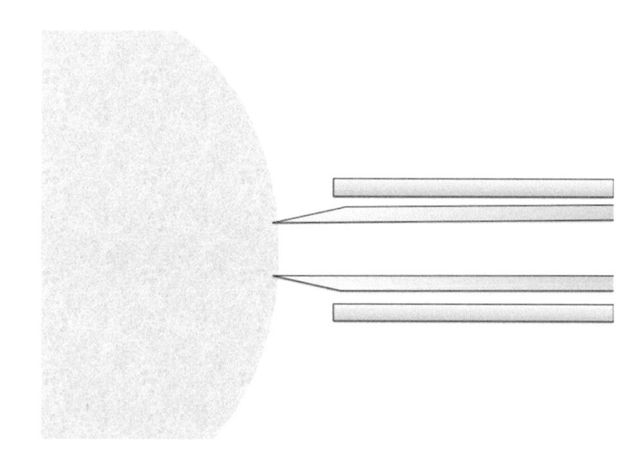

Fig. 6.12 A vibrating blade acting on a malleable tissue only acts push the tissue away from the tip and does not effectively break it down, see below

Fig. 6.13 See Fig. 6.12

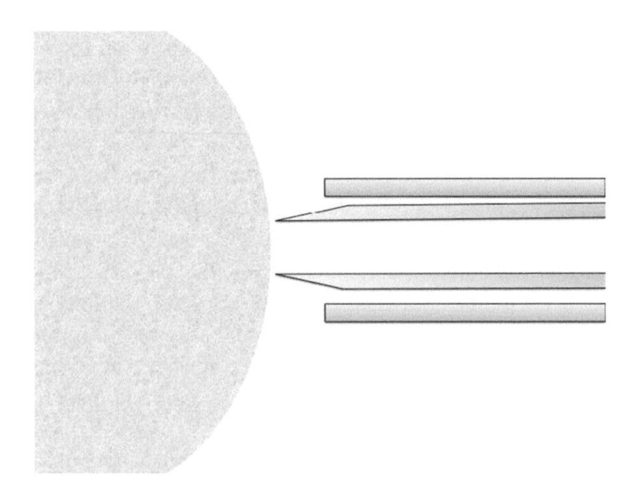

Fig. 6.14 See Fig. 6.12

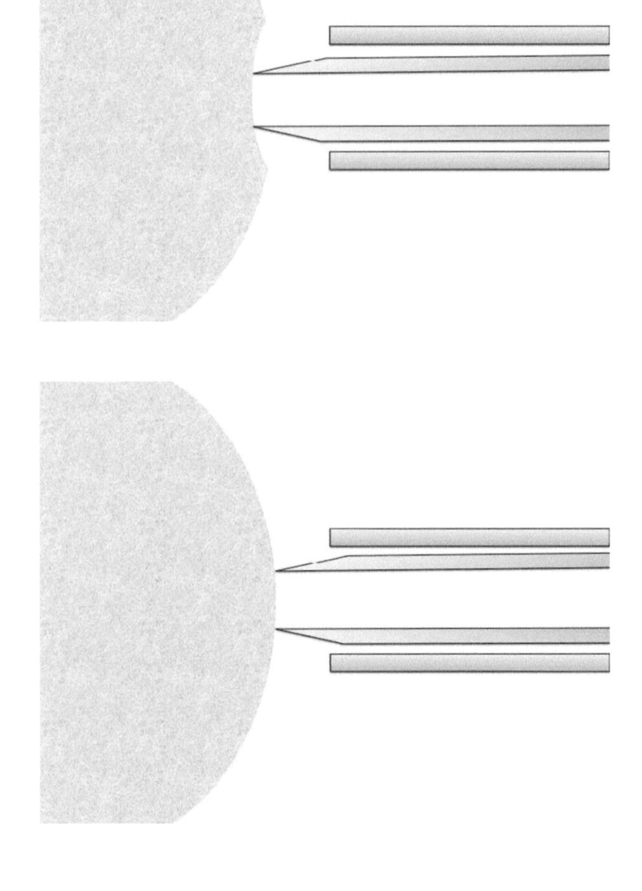

Fig. 6.15 See Fig. 6.12

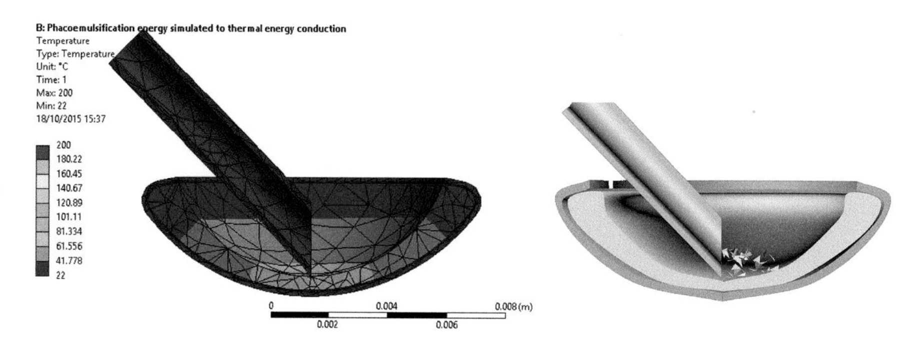

Fig. 6.16 FEA shows phaco-energy simulated to thermal energy. Left shows the pattern of distribution of the thermal energy from the phacoemulsification tip to the lens. Left shows how small lens fragments can be emulsified and vacuumed with minimal contact between the lens the phacoemulsification tip

Fig. 6.17 A guillotine cutter aspirates small segments of a malleable tissue which is sliced off for aspiration by the use of a blade cutting across the orifice, see below

Fig. 6.18 See Fig. 6.17

Fig. 6.19 See Fig. 6.17

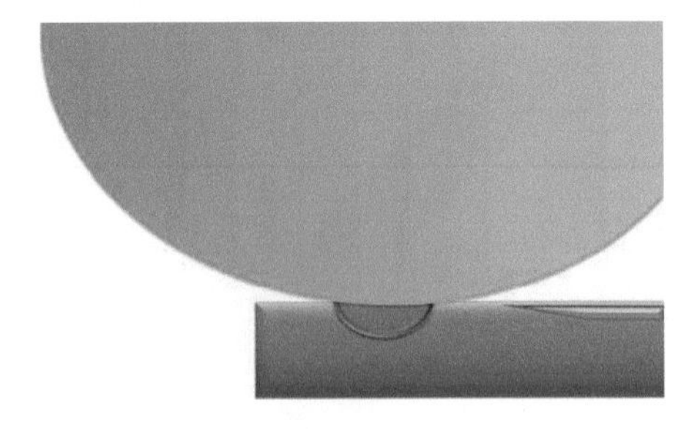

Fig. 6.20 A guillotine cutter cannot engage a hard material unless small fragments are "fed" into the port, see below

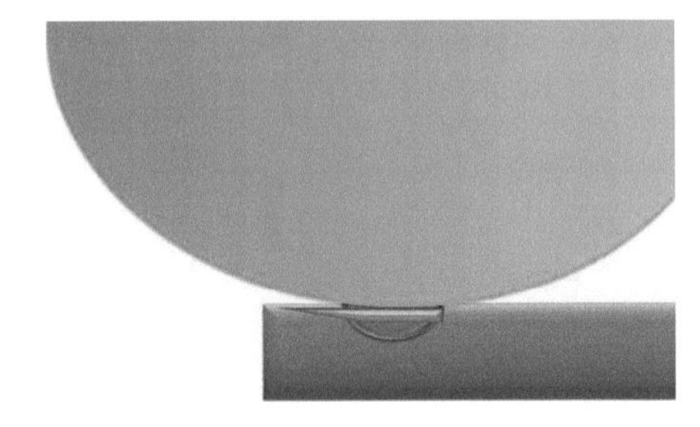

Fig. 6.21 See Fig. 6.20

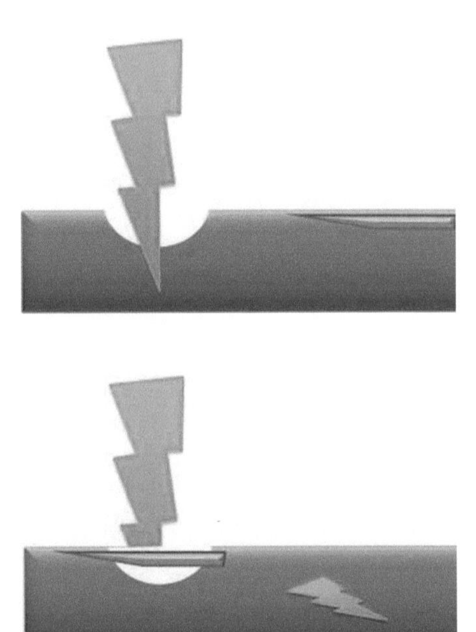

Fig. 6.22 See Fig. 6.20

Fig. 6.23 See Fig. 6.20

Duty Cycle

Duty cycle is a measure of the effectiveness of an instrument. It is determined by the time that the function of the instrument is active over the time period of the function. There may be conditions that maximise the duty cycle for a particular instrument such as port size, speed of oscillations or cutter blades, or the time in which a cutter blade is open or closed.

$$D = \tau / T$$

- D is the duty cycle
- τ is the duration that the function is active
- T is the period of the function

For vitrectomy cutters the larger the caliber of the cutter and the larger the size of the port on the cutter tip, the higher the flow rates that can be achieved. However this is at the cost of a larger wound size for insertion of the instrument. The caliber of cutters is often reduced to 23–27 G to reduce the wound size. Therefore the efficiency of the guillotine becomes more important with increased rates of cuts e.g. 5000 cuts per minute. It is important that there is more time when the orifice is open to aid flow rates and improve the duty cycle. If cut rates are too slow the tissue is less effectively cut because the velocity of the guillotine is less. If the cut rate is too high, the orifice is closed more often than open reducing the flow rate.

References

1. Bond LJ, et al. Physics of phacoemulsification. Washington: United States. Department of Energy; 2003.
2. Fisher R. Elastic constants of the human lens capsule. J Physiol. 1969;201(1):1–19.
3. Weeber HA, et al. Dynamic mechanical properties of human lenses. Exp Eye Res. 2005;80(3):425–34.

Chapter 7
Fluids

Fluids comprise liquids and gases and have particular physical properties that the surgeon can exploit. There are a few physical laws, which are worth understanding and committing to memory, to allow you to fully understand the use of these fluids. The commonest use of a fluid is a balanced salt solution in water (BSS) as an infusion into the eye maintaining the globe volume. However the BSS must flow in tubing and within the eye, which creates physical conditions on the fluid.

It is important to understand some of these conditions.

Flow

- **Flow rate** = Velocity × Cross-sectional Area of the tube
  The flow into the eye will vary with the diameter of the tubing. Similarly, the wound profile and size influence leakage from the wound.

- **Bernoulli's Principle** states that as the speed of a moving liquid increases, the pressure within the liquid decreases. We have looked at this in Chap. 5 in relation to the flow of fluid in an instrument tip.

$$\text{Pressure} \times \text{velocity} = k$$

T.H. Williamson, *Intraocular Surgery: A Basic Surgical Guide*,
DOI 10.1007/978-3-319-27990-9_7

- **Laplace's Law for pressure in a tube radius (r)**

$$\text{Transmural Pressure} = \frac{\text{Wall Tension}}{\text{r}}$$

And a sphere

$$\text{Transmural Pressure} = \frac{2 \times \text{Wall Tension}}{\text{r}}$$

This demonstrates that the larger the fluid filled cavity for the same pressure the higher the tension on the wall. Theoretically a highly myopic eye is more vulnerable to wall rupture for the same pressure inside the eye.

- **Hagan Poiseuille Law**

$$\text{Volume Flow Rate}(\text{Q}) = \frac{\pi \text{d}^4 (\text{Pa} - \text{Pb})}{\text{L8n}}$$

d = diameter of the tube
Pa–Pb = pressure difference between ends
L = length of the tube
n = viscosity

A higher pressure is required to make a highly viscous material such as silicone oil pass through a tube. Flow is increased by the tube's diameter and reduced by its increased length. A high pressure at inflow and low pressure at outflow increase the flow.

- **Reynold's Number**. This is an empirical number to calculate the likelihood of turbulence in a fluid. A thin layer of fluid is unlikely to allow the development of eddies (turbulence).

$$\text{R} = \frac{\text{P2rV}}{\text{N}}$$

R = Reynold's number
P = pressure
r = radius of a tube
n = viscosity of the fluid
V = velocity of the fluid

Therefore a small tube with low velocity fluid under low pressure and with a high viscosity is unlikely to lead to turbulence. However inside the eye where volumes are higher turbulence can occur (Fig. 7.1).

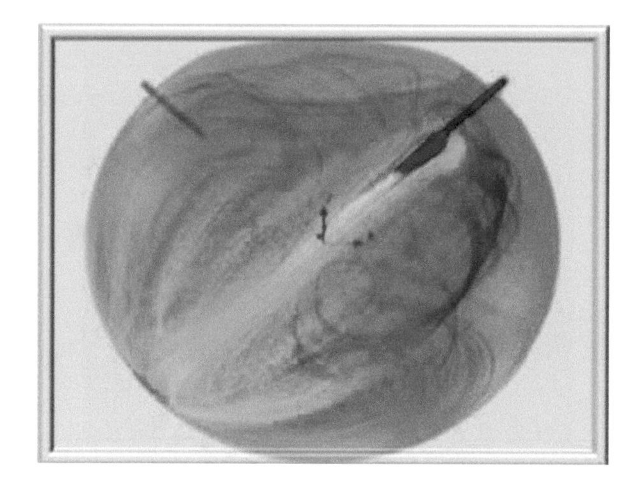

Fig. 7.1 Injecting a fluid into the sphere of the eye creates flow patterns in the eye with possible turbulence (Courtesy of Manoharan Shunmugam)

Viscosity

The viscosity of a fluid is the resistance of a fluid to deformation by a shear stress. Fluids can have Newtonian characteristics where the fluid resists shear flow and strain linearly with time when a stress is applied. In other fluids non-Newtonian properties are seen, where the viscosity increases or decreases with shear rate.

A viscous fluid in elastic tubing, under pressure and in the presence of resistance in the tube, will create tension on the wall of the tube, which will expand the wall. Energy is stored in the expanded wall, which will be transferred to the fluid when the pressure is released causing movement of the fluid down the tube despite release of the pressure in the pump. Similarly when aspirating a viscous fluid with a negative pressure, the wall of the tubing will shrink inwards and return of the wall to its original position we will apply a force to the fluid continuing its extraction despite cessation of the negative pressure at the pump (Figs. 7.2, 7.3 and 7.4).

Viscoelastic Fluids

Some substances exhibit both elastic and viscous properties. These viscoelastic fluids are particularly useful in anterior segment surgery. They have non-Newtonian properties in that the shear stress on the liquid increases with shear rate. The long molecules in the liquid structure give stability to the gel. The gels are resistant to egress from a chamber when rapid deformation is applied. Slower deformations will allow the long molecules to alter their shape. Viscoelastic fluids are therefore used to maintain the space in cavities when rapid deformations might destabilize it whilst allowing instruments to be inserted slowly in and out of the cavity (Figs. 7.5, 7.6, 7.7 and 7.8).

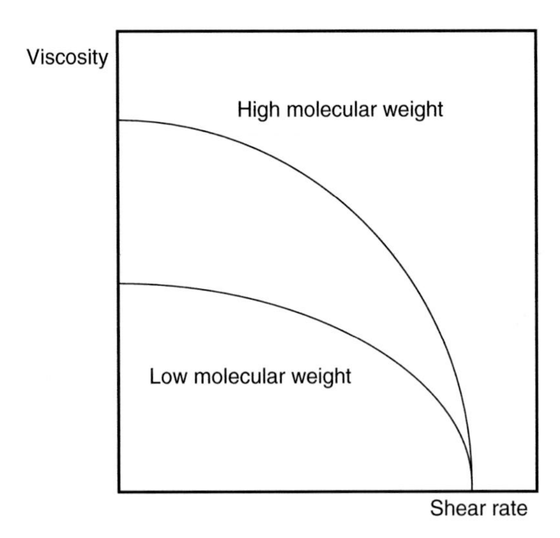

Fig. 7.2 For a visco-elastic structure the viscosity varies with the shear rate. The minimum viscosity depends on the concentration of the molecules in the solution therefore with two substances with similar concentration the curves meet at the lowest viscosity and highest shear rate. The highest viscosity depends upon the molecular weight and therefore the curves separate at high viscosity and low shear rate. At rest the viscosity characteristics of the two fluids are different but both require the same force to inject

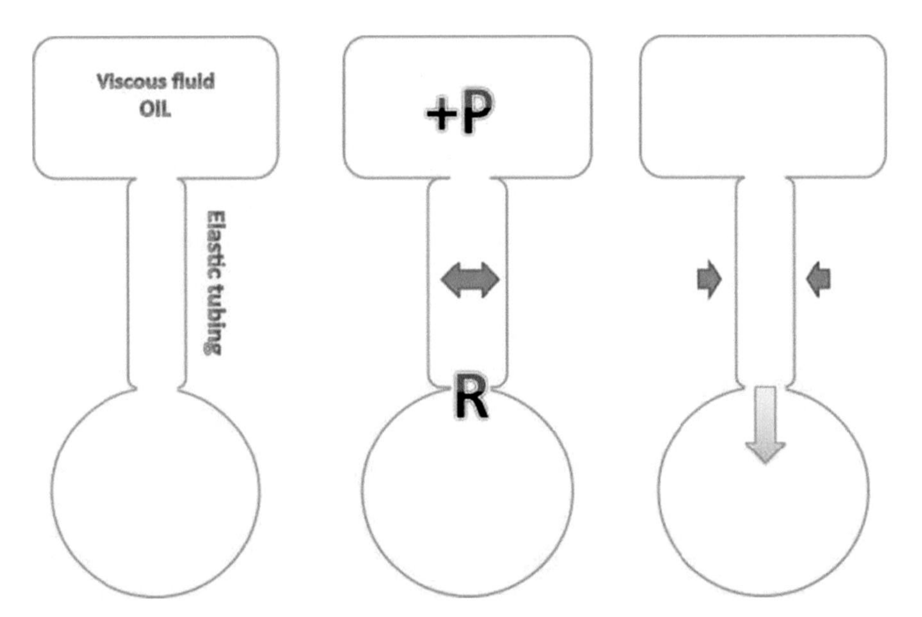

Fig. 7.3 An elastic tubing will expand under pressure given a resistance in the tubing. Once the pressure is released the potential energy in the tube wall causes contraction of the tube and further flow of the fluid in the tube. There is delay before the maximal flow is reached at onset of the pressure and continued flow after the pressure is stopped

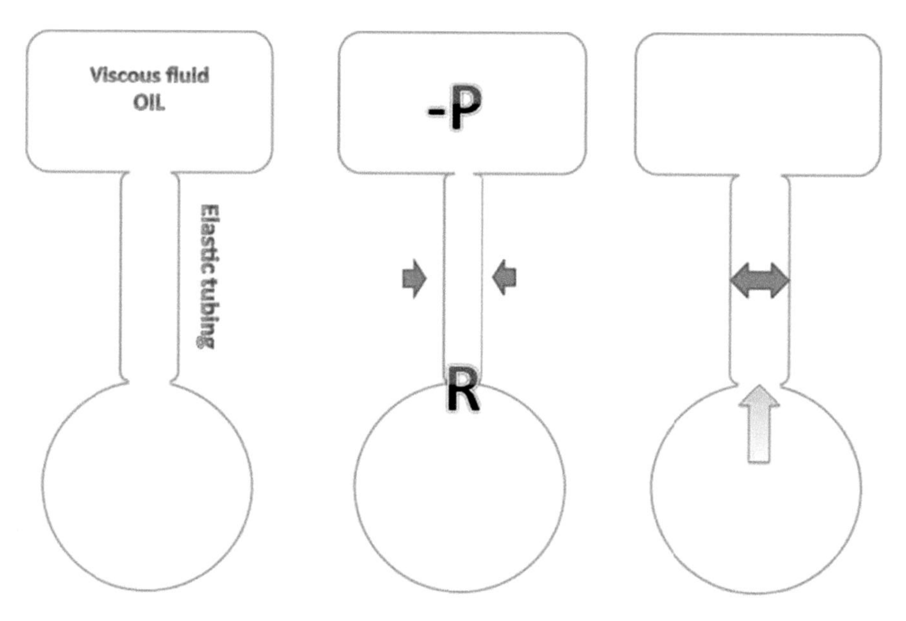

Fig. 7.4 Creating aspiration by negative pressure cause the walls of the tube to contract. On cessation of the negative pressure the walls expand creating flow into the tube after the pressure is stopped

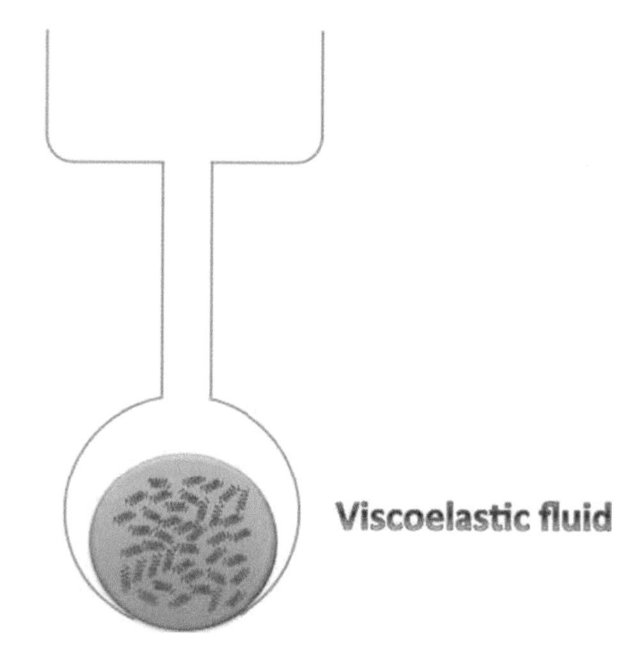

Fig. 7.5 Viscoelastic liquids are used as space fillers to stabilise compartments during surgery

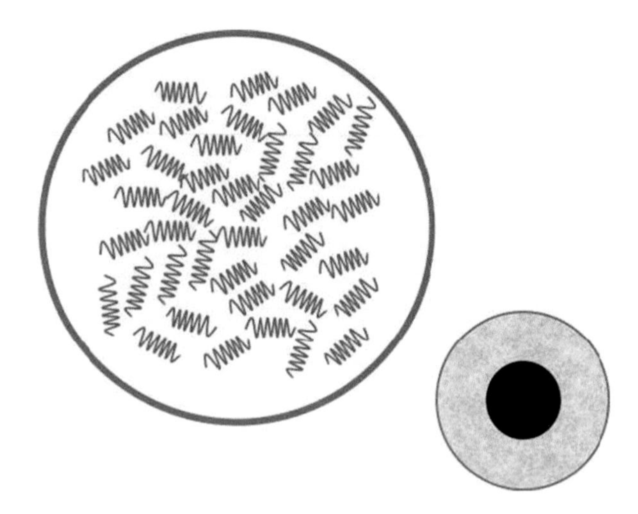

Fig. 7.6 The long chain molecules create a stable gel

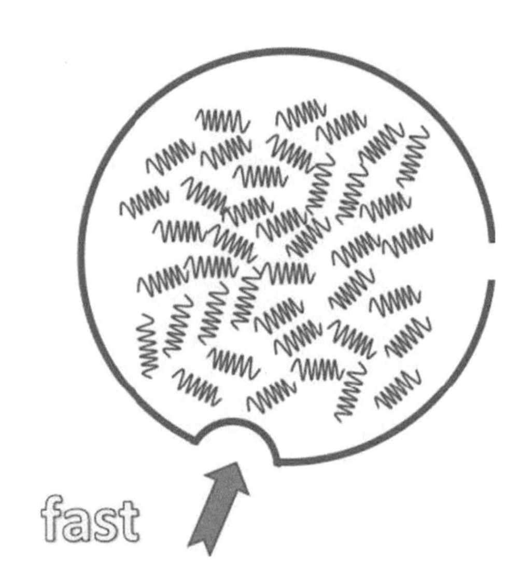

Fig. 7.7 Rapid indentation of the gel does not give the molecules enough time to change shape and the gel structure is preserved (Reprinted from Williamson TH. *Vitreoretinal surgery*, 2nd edition, Springer, 2013)

Diffusion and Convection

Two physical properties are involved in the spread of a pharmaceutical agent in the eye, e.g. intravitreal injections of intra-cameral drugs. These properties are Diffusion and Convection.

- Viscosity is inversely related to diffusion of a molecule
  - Fick's law
    - $\text{Diffusion flux}\left(\text{J}\right) = \text{D} / \text{Concentration gradient}\left(\text{dc} / \text{dx}\right)$

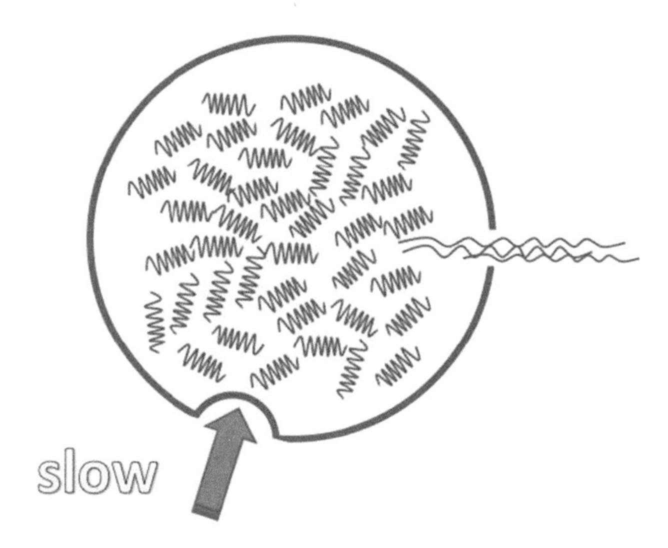

Fig. 7.8 Slow onset indentation allows the molecules to change shape and for the gel to adapt, see below

- Stokes Einstein
  - $\text{Diffusion Coefficient}(D) = RT/6 \;\; nrN$

    D = Diffusion coefficient
    R = Molar gas constant
    T = temperature in Kelvins
    n = viscosity of the medium
    r = radius of the diffusing molecule
    N = Avogadro's number (number of atoms/molecules in one mole of a substance)

Therefore increased temperature and decreased viscosity of the medium increase diffusion.

Convection

- Darcy's law

$$v_{Fluid} = -(K/\mu_{Fluid})P$$

v_{Fluid} = velocity of the fluid
K = hydraulic conductivity
μ_{Fluid} = viscosity of the fluid
P = gradient of pressure

Interfacial Tension

If two liquids come into contact with each other and have different properties preventing them going into solution there may be interactions between the two liquids.

- **Interfacial Tension** exists between two liquids.

Forces are present on the surface of liquid one and liquid two, produced by intermolecular bonds, which must be overcome to break the surface between the two liquids. The interfacial tension in surgery is used to keep a liquid as one bubble, e.g. avoiding the separation off of a bubble, which might pass through for example a wound or a hole in a membrane between compartments. For example, a silicone oil bubble in the eye has a nearly spherical shape because the gravitational forces of the liquid *around* the bubble, which is quite weakly buoyant, are not enough to overcome the interfacial tension of the oil bubble thus giving the natural spherical form. As there is a sphere within a sphere there is much less surface area in contact with the inside of the sphere than with a gas bubble.

Emulsion

This is a complex interaction of otherwise immiscible substances such as oil and water to create small droplets of one in the other. In the eye silicone oil emulsion in aqueous (water) is probably facilitated by the presence of proteins in the aqueous and the mechanical action of eye movements on the surface of the oil bubble. The protein is acting as an emulsifier.

The **Bancroft rule** applies, that is the emulsifiers and emulsifying particles tend to promote dispersion of the phase in which they do not dissolve very well.

The protein dissolves better in water than in oil and so tends to facilitate an oil-in-water emulsion (that is it promotes the dispersion of oil droplets throughout a continuous phase of water).

Evaporation

- **Vapour pressure** is the pressure exerted above a liquid by its own vapour. If a liquid has a high characteristic vapour pressure then the liquid is more likely to evaporate.

Some fluids used in surgery such as perfluorocarbons are easily converted into a gaseous state because they have a high vapour pressure. Therefore if an air bubble is inserted in the presence of these liquids small droplets may evaporate into the air.

- **Liquids are not compressible for practical purposes;** this means that the liquid cannot absorb deformations in the eye during surgery. There must be a flow of the liquid out of the eye either from the wound or up the infusion tubing.

- **Pascal's Principle,** Pressure is transmitted undiminished in an enclosed static fluid. Therefore a movement of fluid is transmitted to the opposite wall of a compartment.

Gases

Air bubbles and large molecule gases are used in ocular surgery as per-operative tools or for their properties in the postoperative period.

In contrast to liquids, gases are compressible. Often there is an interaction with the gas and surrounding liquids.

- **Surface Tension**. The forces are present on the surface of a liquid and a gas, produced by intermolecular bonds, which must be overcome to break the surface of the liquid in gas.
  - The surface tension in surgery is used to keep the gas as one bubble, e.g. avoiding the separation off of a bubble
  - An air or gas bubble in the eye has a flattened inferior aspect because the gravitational force of the liquid under the bubble, combined with the high buoyancy of the gas, is strong enough to overcome the surface tension of the gas bubble (which without gravitational forces would create a sphere), thus causing the bubble to flatten inferiorly rather than achieve a sphere. Similarly the forces acting on the bubble are enough to overcome the surface tension to cause the bubble to conform to the shape of the sphere (the eye) superiorly.
  - As the bubble becomes smaller the balance of gravitational forces relative to surface tension is changed. If a bubble separates off, it remains so because the surface tension effects overcome the gravitational effects of the fluid and the fluid remains between the bubbles separating them, therefore multiple separate bubbles appear just before the bubble disperses (Fig. 7.9).
- **Fick's Diffusion equation** states that the rate of diffusion of a gas through a thin membrane is increased by: the concentration differential; area of the membrane; the diffusivity of the gas and reduced by the thickness of the membrane. This equation explains the longevity of some large molecule gases e.g. perfluoropropane, in the eye, and why these can expand.

$$F = -D(c2 - c1)/x$$

- F = rate of passage of the gas
- D = diffusivity of the gas
- c2–c1 = gas concentration difference across the membrane
- x = thickness of thin membrane (Fig. 7.10)
- **Boyle's law** states that, at a constant temperature, the volume of a given mass of gas varies inversely with pressure

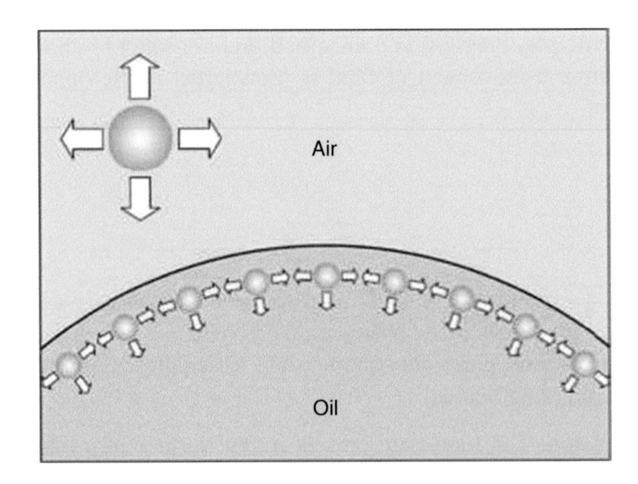

Fig. 7.9 The intermolecular attractions are shown around the molecules in a liquid (e.g. oil) in contact with another liquid or a gas (e.g. air). Within the liquid each molecule is pulled equally in all directions by neighbouring liquid molecules top left, resulting in a net force of zero. At the surface of the liquid, the molecules are more attracted to other molecules inside the liquid than outside in the gas, producing an overall force inwards. The liquid would like to be a sphere but is usually distorted by other forces e.g. gravitational (Reprinted from Williamson TH. *Vitreoretinal surgery*, 2nd edition, Springer, 2013)

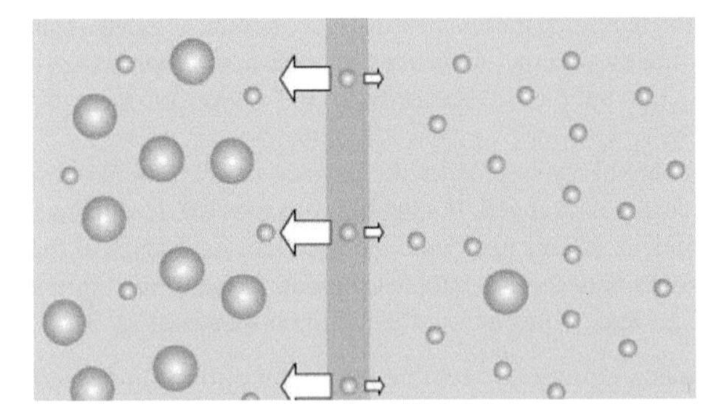

Fig. 7.10 Gases molecules separated by a semi-permeable membrane will move across the membrane until they have reached equilibrium. A large molecule gas has low diffusivity and passes across the membrane slowly. A small molecule gas moves rapidly across the membrane. Therefore initially the gas bubble on the left expands in relation to the gas bubble on the right (Reprinted from Williamson TH. *Vitreoretinal surgery*, 2nd edition, Springer, 2013)

Chapter 8
Microscopes, Light and Lasers

The commonest source of illumination for ocular surgery is the microscope light. Systems may employ Halogen, Xenon or LED sources of light.

Field of View and Magnification

Visualisation can be influenced by the field of view provided by the equipment and the quality of the image (dependent upon the degradation of the image by the optical elements of the instrument). Field of view is reduced when increased magnification is used. If magnification is increased then field of view is decreased. The advantages to a surgical manoeuvre from the introduction of high magnification can be lost because the reduced field of view creates other problems such as the potential for unnoticed damage to peripheral tissues. Manoeuvres may be performed best with a balance of magnification and field of view.

If a variable aperture is available this should be adjusted until the smallest aperture is reached at which the illumination is not noticeably reduced. This will maximise the depth of focus of the image in the same way that the photographer uses a small aperture to increase depth of focus in a photograph.

During illumination from the operating microscope, retro-illumination of structures is provided by a co-axial light (or light slightly angled at 2°), which shines through the pupil of the eye. This provides better contrast for certain manoeuvres during surgery.

Light hazard to the retina varies with wavelength of the light with shorter wavelengths more hazardous. Filters may be used in the light source to remove the blue or ultraviolet spectrum. Tissue damage increases with illumination and duration of exposure to light in addition therefore lower illumination and shorter duration of surgery are both useful.

T.H. Williamson, *Intraocular Surgery: A Basic Surgical Guide*,
DOI 10.1007/978-3-319-27990-9_8

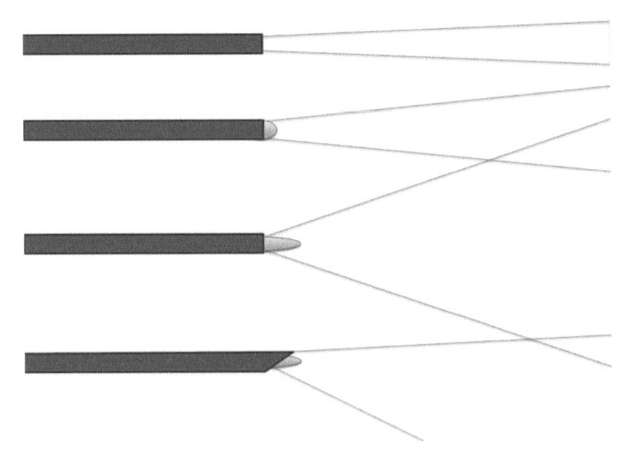

Fig. 8.1 Fibre optic lights can be used to illuminate the inside of the eye. Depending on the profile of the tip of the fibre optic light can be localised, diffuse or eccentric

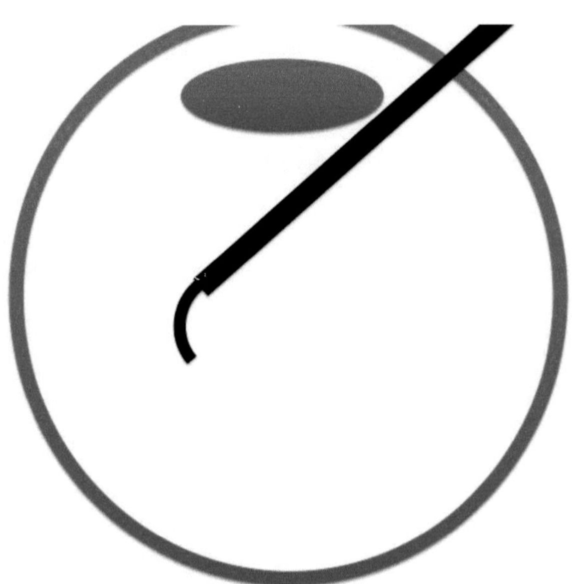

Fig. 8.2 Applying a curve to the fibre optic is useful if applying laser. This allows the surgeon to apply the laser at 90° to the surface to be treated maintaining a focused treatment area

Fibre Optics

Fibre optic instruments can be used to provide light inside the sphere of the eye. The tips of the fibre optic can be varied to provide different angles of illumination (Figs. 8.1, 8.2, 8.3, 8.4, 8.5, 8.6 and 8.7).

Laser

Laser is an acronym for "light amplification by stimulated emission of radiation". It is the coherence of the light from the laser both temporally and spatially, which give it the properties allowing aiming and focussing of the light energy.

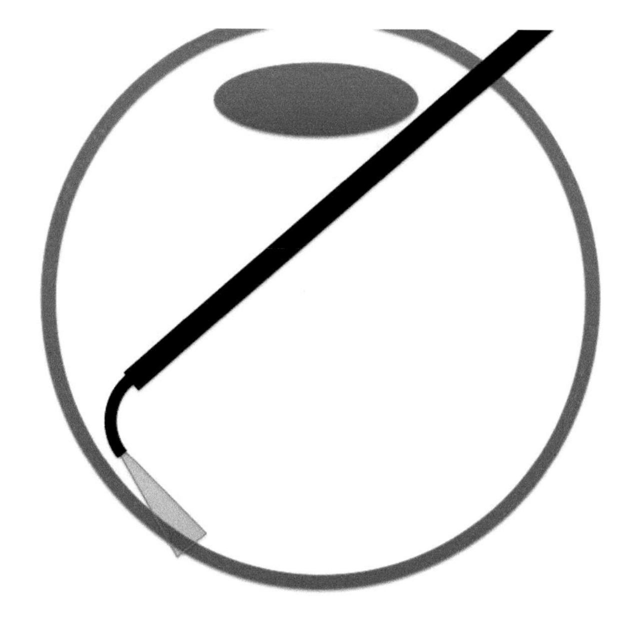

Fig. 8.3 Applying the laser obliquely to the surface creates a diffuse burn which is elongated and difficult to control

Fig. 8.4 Some fibre optics can be retracted up the sleeve of the instrument to vary the curvature

Types of laser in ophthalmology:

- Argon is a laser with ionized argon as the active medium and with a beam in the blue and green visible light spectrum; used for photocoagulation.
- Excimer laser (excited dimer) is a laser with rare gas halides as the active medium. The laser is in the ultraviolet spectrum. Its effect is to break chemical bonds without heat and with minimal penetration of tissues.
- Neodymium:yttrium-aluminum-garnet (Nd:YAG) laser has a medium of a crystal of yttrium, aluminum, and garnet doped with neodymium ions. The laser is

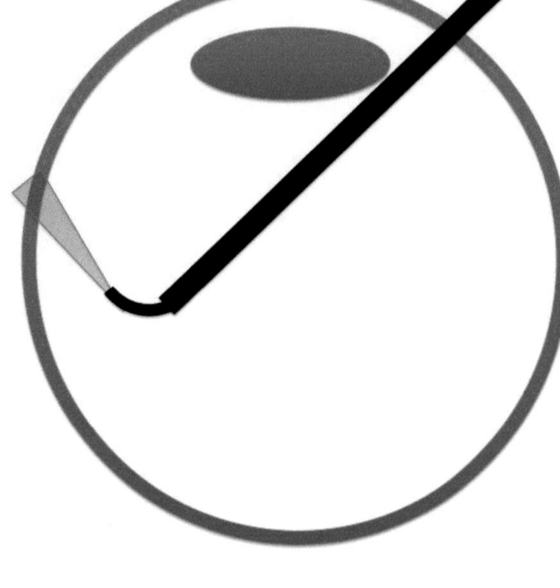

Fig. 8.5 The curve aids reaching the whole internal surface, important as the entry point of the fibre optic is fixed

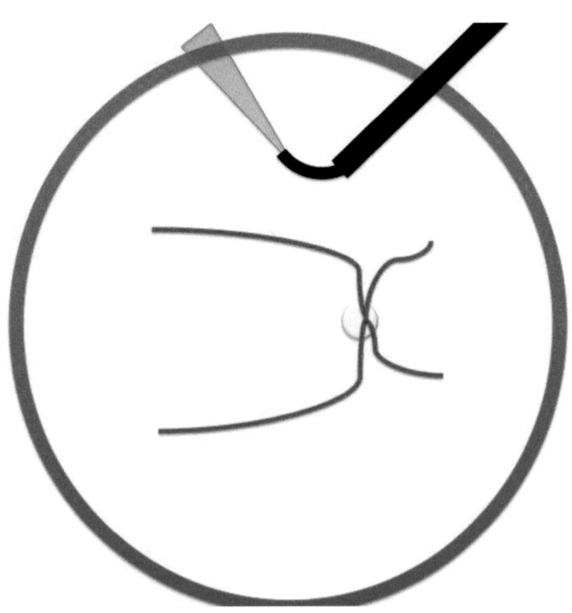

Fig. 8.6 The curve allows the application of laser in different directions whilst maintaining 90°

near infrared spectrum at approximately 1060 nm and can be used for photocoagulation and photoablation.

Argon lasers (514 nm wavelength), double frequency YAG lasers (532 nm), dye lasers (577–630 nm), diode pumped solid-state lasers (532 nm) and diode lasers are available. Argon provides wavelengths in the blue and green spectra but has been

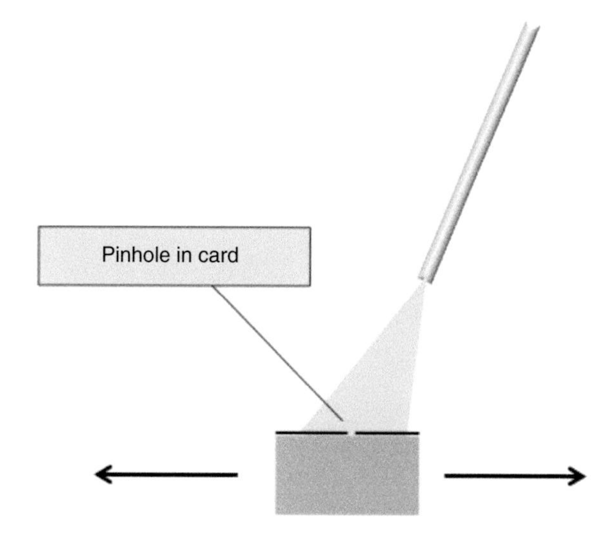

Fig. 8.7 The light intensity increases as the light is closer to the tissue and in the centre of the beam

recently superseded by others such as double frequency YAG laser (producing a 532 nm wavelength from a YAG tube, normally 1064 nm), partly because manufacturers can produce smaller more portable equipment of higher reliability.

Laser is focussed to achieve the desired effect usually a thermal burn. The thermal burn consists of protein denaturation and coagulation at 60 °C seen as blanching of the tissue (photocoagulation). It can be difficult to titrate the dose of irradiation as the desired effect is non linear. A threshold must be reached before the desired effect can be seen. Therefore the surgeon must gradually increase the laser parameters until the minimum is reached to achieve an effect. The lowest power to achieve a visible effect indicates to the user the threshold at which an effect is gained without side effects. If the temperature is raised too high, to 100 °C, the water in the tissue boils, expanding into a gas. This creates cavitation and cell rupture. Loss of the water creates a rapid temperature rise and at 300 °C the tissue can carbonise.

The photons from laser scatter within the biological tissues and create an spheroidal spread. Therefore the burn produced is wider than the diameter of the laser light and there is scatter of energy anteriorly and even more so posteriorly from the point of focus of the laser. Short duration, high power laser application creates a long narrow area of damage from scatter. Long duration, low power laser application creates a shallower but wider area of damage and the thermal energy has time to spread by conduction (Figs. 8.8 and 8.9).

Different wavelengths of laser have different effects on tissue. As wavelength shortens the absorption increases and the scatter decreases. On the retina, in the green spectrum a thermal burn is produced in the retinal pigment epithelium, easily identified by whitening of the tissue. It is therefore easy to adjust the dosage to produce the minimum burn necessary for adhesion or controlled damage of the retina without damaging superficial retinal nerve fibres causing further visual loss. Yellow lasers (561 nm) are available which may have advantages around the macula because

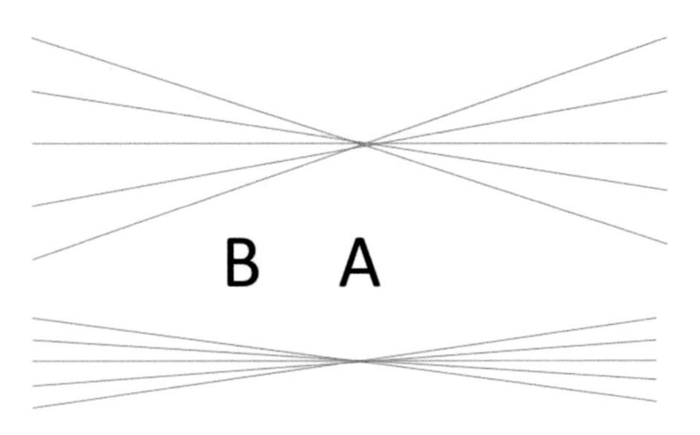

Fig. 8.8 For laser to create a burn the laser is focussed at point A. The more diffuse the spread of laser before or after the focal point the less chance of tissue effects away from the focal point, B (Reprinted from Williamson TH. *Vitreoretinal Surgery*, 2nd edition, Springer, 2013)

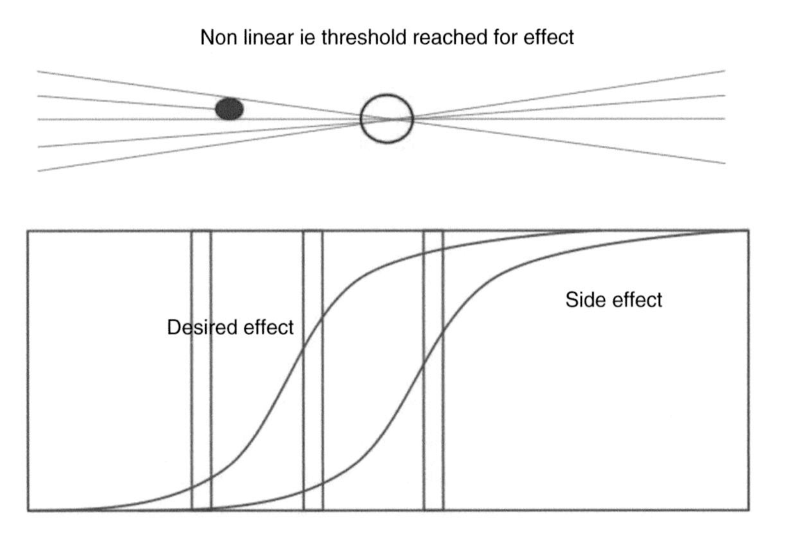

Fig. 8.9 Laser creates its thermal effect when a threshold of energy is reached. The surgeon needs to gradually increase the energy until the effect is seen but is not provided with information from the tissue reaction until that point. Starting with a high energy setting risks moving into the side effect portion of the treatment profile

of reduced absorption by Xanthophyll. Diode lasers are available which produce a wavelength of 810 nm (infrared), these burn deep into the retina and choroid without a visible burn on the retina until a large burn has occurred in the choroid. Care must be taken when using diode lasers that choroidal ischemia is not created.

As the tissue is altered by the thermal energy the absorption and scatter properties are changed. The initial burn may increase posterior scattering until the tissue carbonises when anterior scattering increases.

Most often laser is applied using a slit lamp and various contact lenses. The optics of these lenses may alter the effects of the laser by magnification (Tables 8.1 and 8.2).

Table 8.1 Laser effects may be altered by viewing lenses

Lens	Viewing (image) magnification	Laser spot magnification
Ocular Mainster PRP 165	×0.51	×1.96
Volk SuperQuad 160	×0.5	×2.0
Volk equator plus	×0.44	×2.27
Goldmann 3-mirror	×1.06	~ ×0.94

Table 8.2 Absorption of laser wavelengths

	Laser Wavelength		
Chromophore	Green (514–532 nm)	Yellow (560–580 nm)	Red (620–676)
Melanin	High	High	Moderate
Oxygenated Haemoglobin	High	High	Low
Reduced Haemoglobin	High	High	Moderate
Xanthophyll	Minimal	Negligible	Negligible

Yag Laser

Nd:YAG (Neodymium-Doped Yttrium Aluminium Garnet; Nd:$Y_3Al_5O_{12}$)

Nd:YAG lasers are examples of solid state lasers because they use laser diode to pump a solid crystal (Nd:YAG crystal) which produces an emission wavelength of 1064 nm (infrared). The wavelength can be frequency doubled to provide a "green" laser for photocoagulation.

In ophthalmology the laser can be operated in Q-switch mode. In this modality, the usual return of light into the medium is prevented during activation of the medium by the diode laser. When maximal energy is reached in the medium the light is allowed to return causing a very short (nanoseconds) and very high release of energy (kilowatts). The high energy causes ionization of atoms and plasma formation, i.e. atoms stripped of electrodes, with a surrounding area of high pressure (creating a destructive shock wave) when applied to the tissue.

These lasers are used to disrupt tissues, which can be reached through optically clear media without the need for the tissue to absorb the wavelength of the laser. They are used on relatively transparent tissues such a posterior capsules in lens implants or the cornea (intralase). They may be used on tissues where a thermal burn would be undesirable such as peripheral iris.

Chapter 9
Suturing

In most circumstances sutures are used to appose the surfaces of a wound to allow the wound to heal more rapidly and without ingress of granulation tissue. In the fluid filled eye the sutures compress surfaces of the wound together to avoid leakage of fluid from the eye. The diameter of the sutures in ophthalmology is very small and therefore the surgeon usually holds the suture with micro forceps. The first thing to learn is how to hold a suture with instruments. It is important not to stress the suture, which might cause breakage, for this reason the orientation of a forceps to the suture is important. Any attempt to angle the surfaces of the forceps at 90° to the suture should be resisted as this may snap the suture, it is better to allow a suture to remain straight and use the friction of the two opposed surfaces to hold the suture (Fig. 9.1).

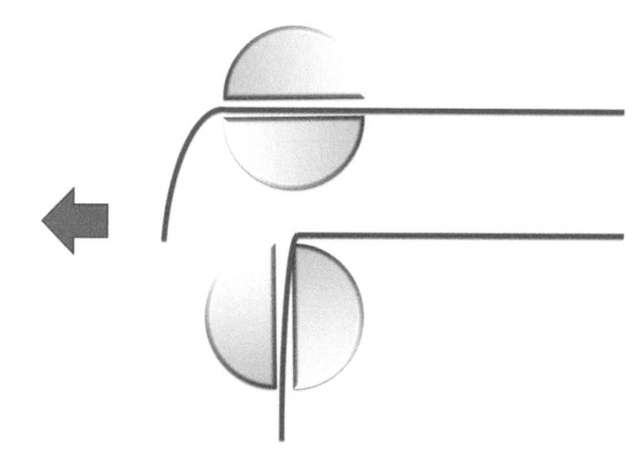

Fig. 9.1 When holding a suture in forceps keep the surfaces of the forceps parallel to the pull on the suture. Angling the forceps risks snapping the suture at the junction of the suture

T.H. Williamson, *Intraocular Surgery: A Basic Surgical Guide*,
DOI 10.1007/978-3-319-27990-9_9

Single Sutures

Sutures are usually connected to the needle by wrapping the metal of the needle around the suture. This creates a cylindrical shape at the end of the needle. Elsewhere the needle will have different profiles depending on the suture track being created. In most circumstances in ophthalmology the main shaft of the needle is flattened to allow the needle track to be flat rather than round. When holding the needle place the forceps on the main shaft of the needle where it is flattened, this stabiles the needle in the forceps. Holding the needle at its cylindrical end is less stable and risks rotation of the needle during usage.

The ideal suture track to provide closure of a wound would possess a circular profile through the wound, however this is impossible to achieve in the small structures of the eye. Any eccentricity of the circle to the wound will distort the tissues because the superficial tissue is forced to move downwards and the interior wound opens (Fig. 9.2).

In practice, a semicircular suture track profile with entry and exit points on the surface of the tissue at 90° and deep insertion of the wound to nearly 100 % of the tissue provides best closure. Inserting to 100 % creates a potential track for leakage and infection from the internal to the external surface (Fig. 9.3).

Unfortunately the creation of a needle with the same radius as this semi-circular suture track will cause the needle to be lost within the wound. Therefore the surgeon cannot access the needle. In practice, the needle must have a greater radius of curvature than the desired track so that the forceps can grip the needle. The needle is inserted by distorting the wound during its insertion; everting the wound as the needle is inserted creates the correct wound profile (Fig. 9.4).

A wound may be distorted by over-tightening of the suture because over-tightening of the suture causes the suture track to take on a more spherical profile. This again creates problems by forcing the external wound downwards whilst opening up the internal wound (Figs. 9.5, 9.6 and 9.7)

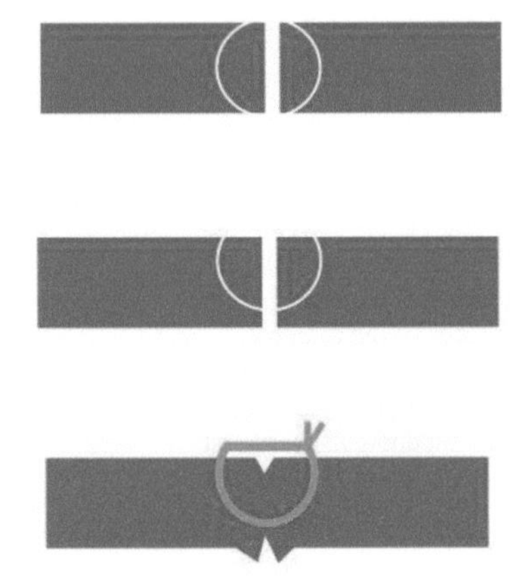

Fig. 9.2 *Top*, an ideal suture profile but not achievable in thin structures. *Middle*, an eccentric circle distorts the tissue on tightening, *bottom*

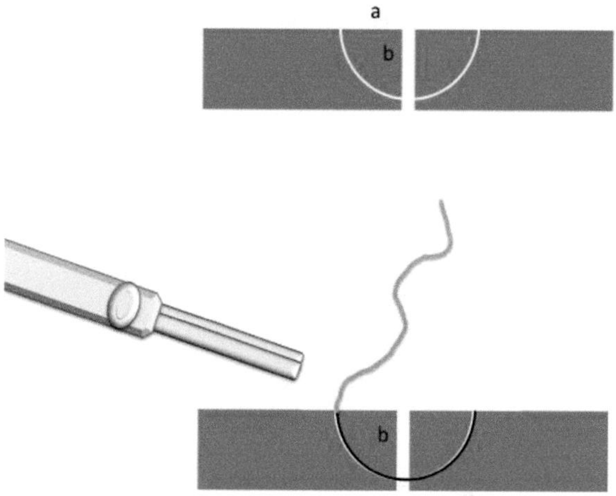

Fig. 9.3 A needle of the exact curve of the suture track is difficult to manipulate in the track

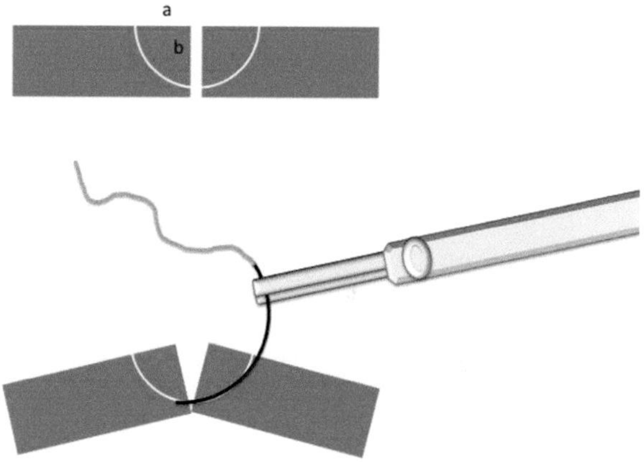

Fig. 9.4 It is commoner to use a needle with a shallower curve and distort the tissue on insertion to increase the curvature of the track

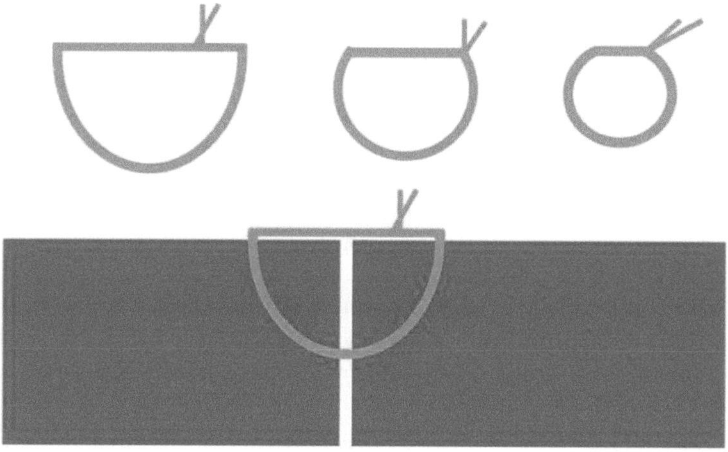

Fig. 9.5 Over tightening of a suture causes the suture to become more circular in profile

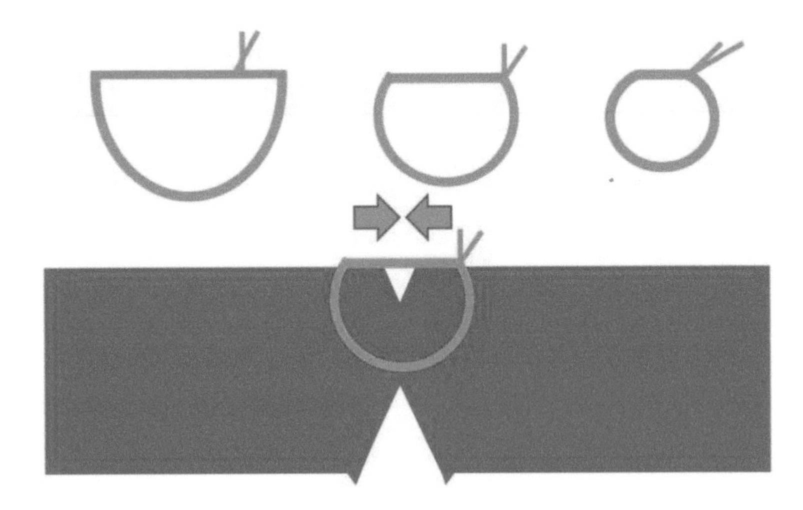

Fig. 9.6 A tight shallow suture causes gaping of the interior wound edges

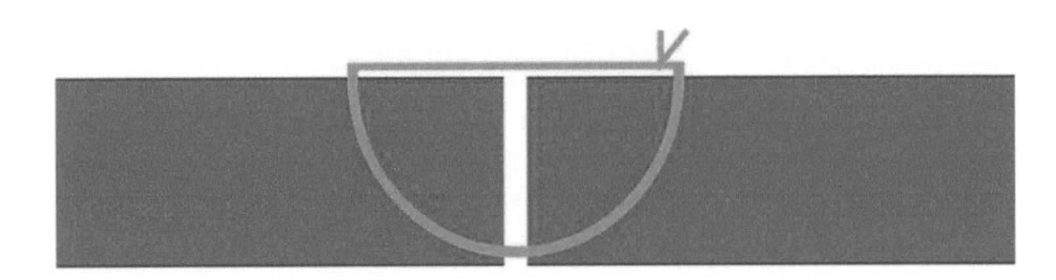

Fig. 9.7 The ideal suture is as deep as possible without penetrating the tissue layer, passes into and out of the tissue at 90° and through the wound at 90° at an equal depth. The tension is enough to close but not to distort the tissue

A suture track, which is too shallow, increases the chance of gaping of the internal wound. In contrast a deep track with 90° exit and entry of the suture and the correct tension on the suture creates good apposition of the surfaces of the wound.

Oblique wounds are more difficult to close because tension on the tissue can compress the wound edge distorting the wound. It is useful to have the suture passed through the wound at 90° to prevent movement of the wound and this can be achieved by moving the suture closer to the external wound site.

Restricting the closure to the superficial tissue can close a stepped wound; however over-tightening at this site will cause the internal orifice to open (Figs. 9.8, 9.9, 9.10 and 9.11).

We have seen before how a shelved wound will only open if a line joining the external corners of the external wound crosses over the arc of the internal wound. A simple suture placed on the external wound creates another focal point through which the crossing lining can pass. In this way a long wound is turned into two small wounds, which restores the integrity of the wound. Sutures can in this way

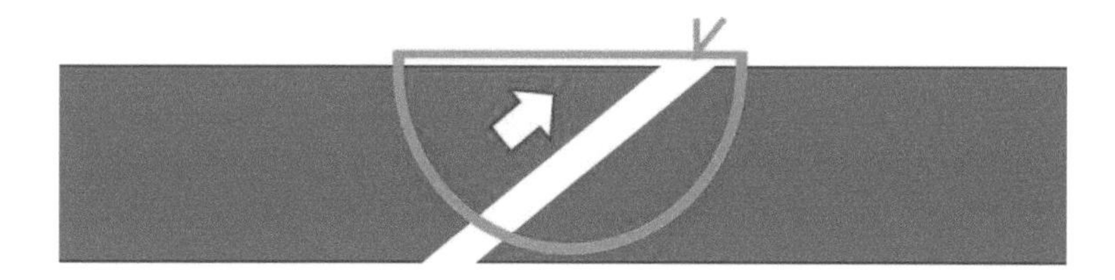

Fig. 9.8 Suturing an oblique wound risks sliding of the wound if the suture does not pass at a right angle through the incision

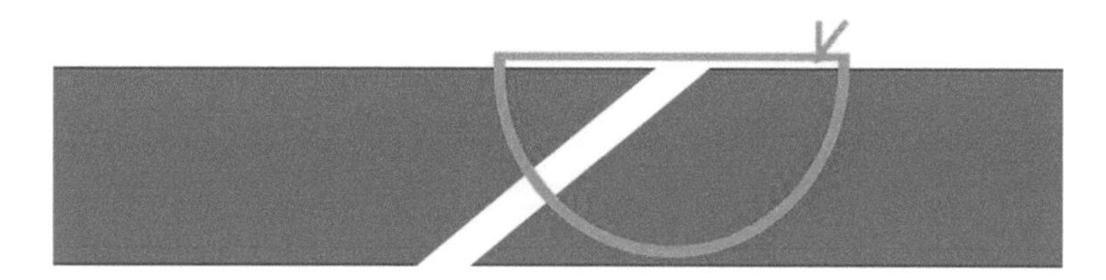

Fig. 9.9 See Fig. 9.8

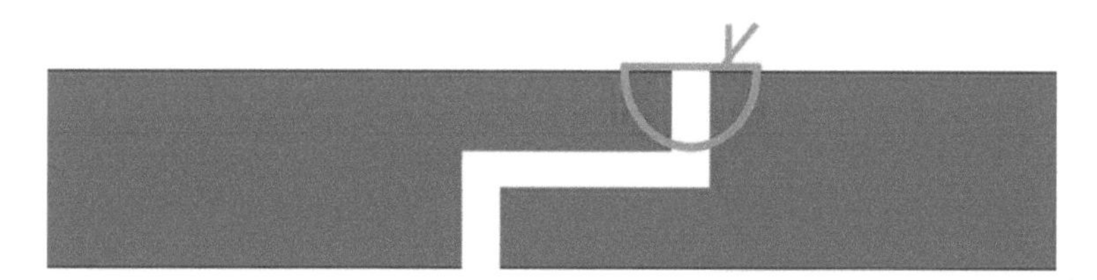

Fig. 9.10 A stepped wound can be closed by suturing the outer flap only

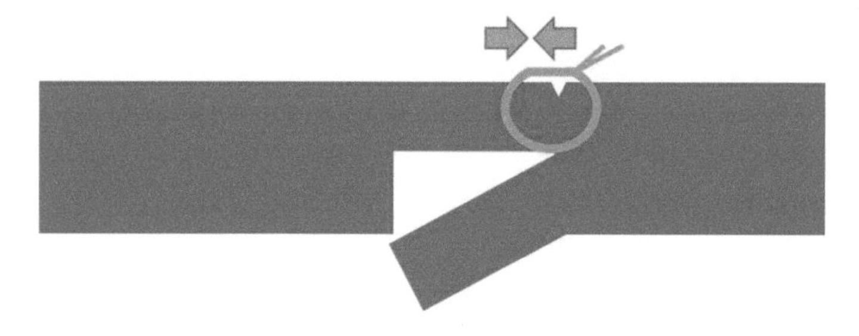

Fig. 9.11 Over tightening the outer suture can distort the inner wound

restore a wound's integrity without the need for excessive numbers of stitches (Figs. 9.12 and 9.13).

Inserting sutures on a curved surface can have the effect of flattening that surface because a suture with tension will try and achieve a profile in one plane. A circular

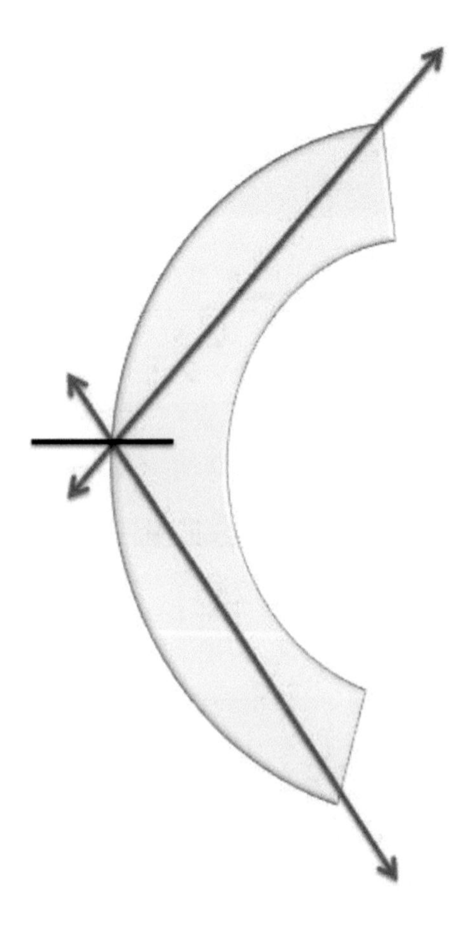

Fig. 9.12 Inserting a suture changes a shelved wound into two smaller shelved wounds. This prevents leakage because a line between the suture and the corner of the external wound does not pass over the internal wound

suture under tension will form a flat circle with the effect that it will flatten the surface. A zigzag suture once tightened will straighten and flatten the surface (Fig. 9.14).

Continuous Sutures

Continuous sutures are useful in that they spread the load of compression over the area covered by the suture, whereas it can be difficult to get the same tension on all of a group of interrupted sutures. Although the continuous suture compresses the wound in the desired direction (perpendicular to the wound), there are secondary effects e.g. also compressing the wound parallel to the wound. The latter is usually an undesirable effect on the wound as it shortens the length of the tissue (Fig. 9.15).

To minimise distortion of a tissue by a continuous suture, the width of each suture bite needs to be equal. Larger bites over the course of a continuous suture will create a greater effect resulting in compression of the tissue excessively where the large bite is located (Fig. 9.16).

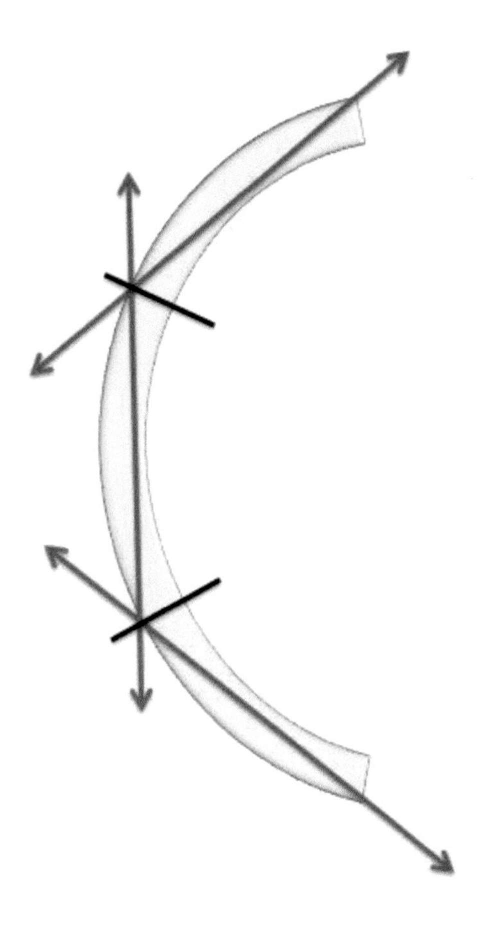

Fig. 9.13 For longer wounds the wound can be segmented by carefully placed sutures

Ragged wounds can be sutured with continuous suture but because of the different actions of this suture the position of the bites relative to the wound should be varied to allow the suture to have a symmetrical profile. Alternatively the ragged wound can be sutured with in the interrupted sutures in which case each one needs to be at 90° to the wound wherever its place. For triangulated wounds, in order to keep tension on the apex of the triangle the orientation of the interrupted sutures should be angled progressively towards the apex (Figs. 9.17 and 9.18).

Curved wounds are common in ophthalmology, and require specific approaches to their closure. Again interrupted sutures should be kept at 90° to the wound at the site of the insertion. Continuous sutures must be angulated appropriate to the position on the curve. Continuous sutures will have secondary effects of trying to straighten out the curve when placed under tension (Figs. 9.19 and 9.20).

Long interrupted sutures spread the force of the compression over a larger area, and therefore a reduced number of sutures are required. Short sutures spread the compressive force over a small area and therefore more sutures are required. A tight suture will spread its force further laterally. Placement of the suture in an oblong fashion to the wound causes the wound surfaces to want to move to allow the suture

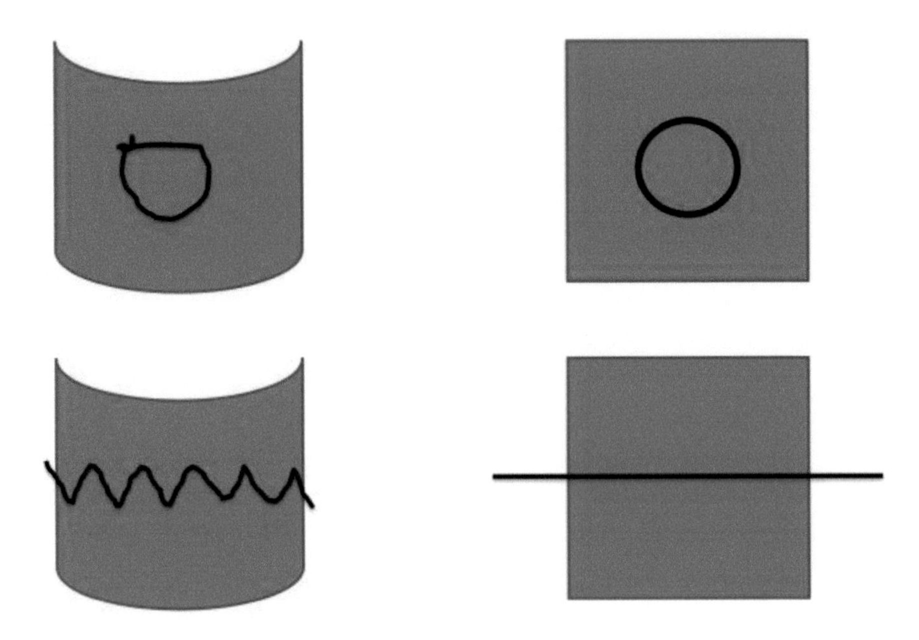

Fig. 9.14 Tight sutures will try to flatten the plane in which they lie. A circular or continuous suture will flatten a curved surface

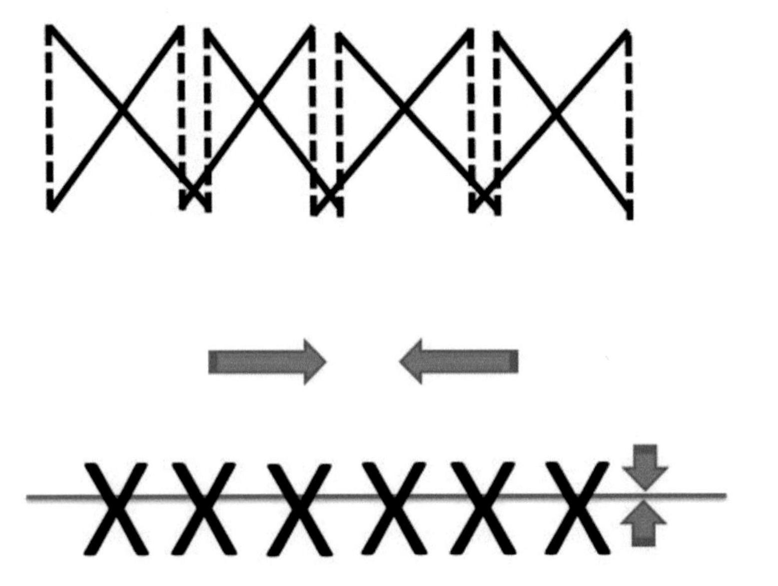

Fig. 9.15 A continuous suture will contract a wound in a direction parallel to the wound

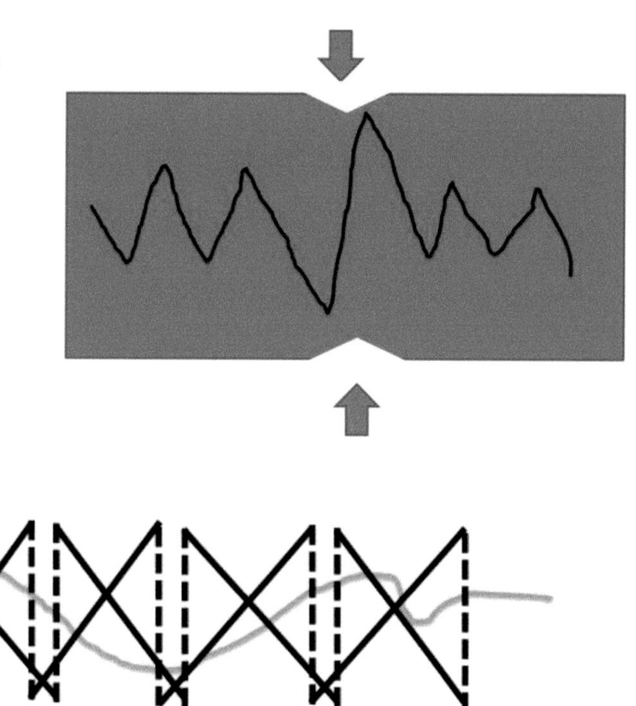

Fig. 9.16 An irregularly spaced continuous suture will cause variable contraction of tissue

Fig. 9.17 A ragged wound can be sutured with continuous suture thus

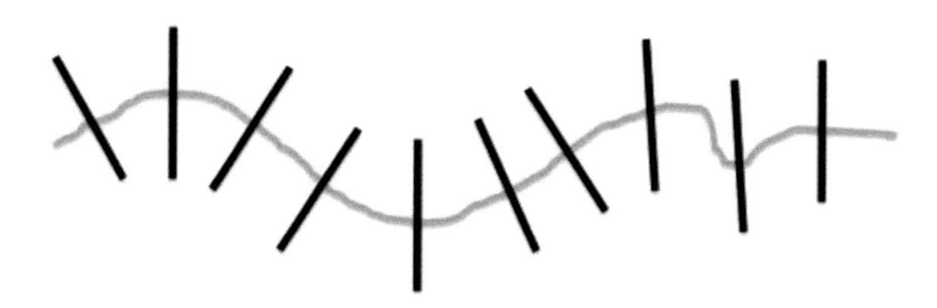

Fig. 9.18 Interrupted sutures can be used to close a ragged wound but should be perpendicular to the wound at insertion

to become 90° to the wound. This potentially distorts the wound and is usually undesirable (Figs. 9.21, 9.22 and 9.23).

Sutures also have effects in 3 dimensions, for example continuous sutures depress and elevate tissue within the wound under tension. In general, interrupted sutures have less distorting effects if placed carefully as the depressing and elevating forces are aligned. The single suture with two bites will cause depression of the tissue at the location of the external suture and elevation of the tissue where the sutures internally placed, again because the suture wants to exist on the same plane (Figs. 9.24, 9.25 and 9.26)

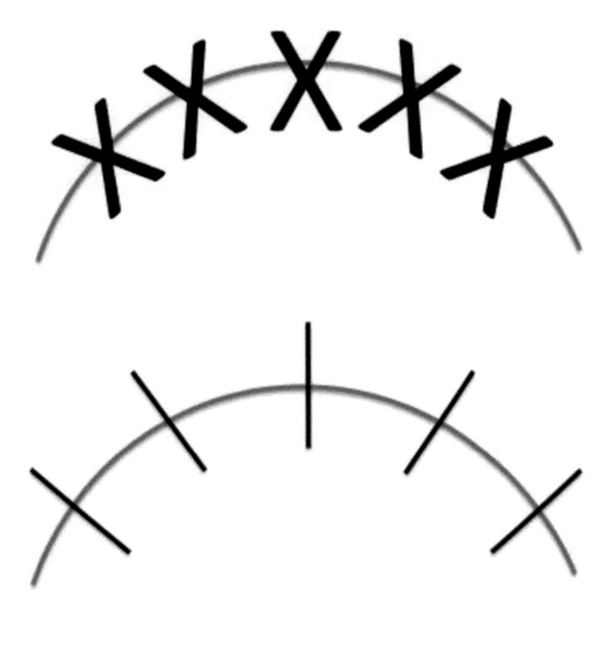

Fig. 9.19 A continuous suture has the advantage of spreading an even force over the wound. In contrast the tension on interrupted sutures must be individually adjusted

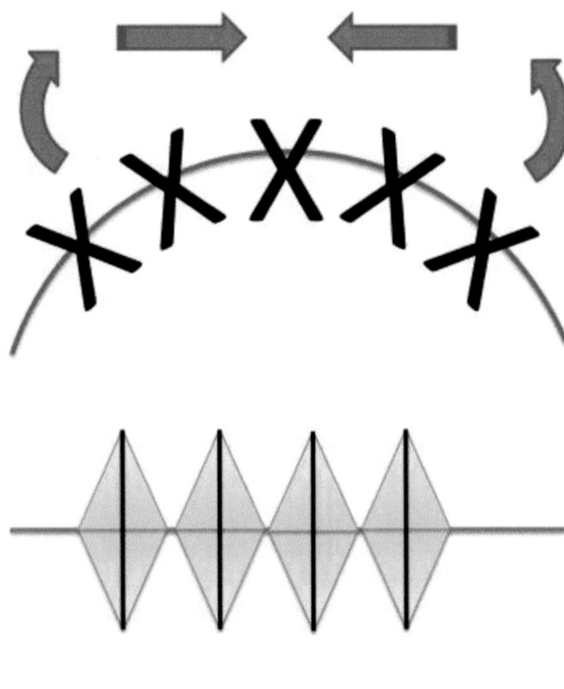

Fig. 9.20 The continuous suture will try to straighten the curved wound when under tension

Fig. 9.21 A compression suture spreads the force in a triangular fashion with longer sutures providing and wider spread than shorter ones

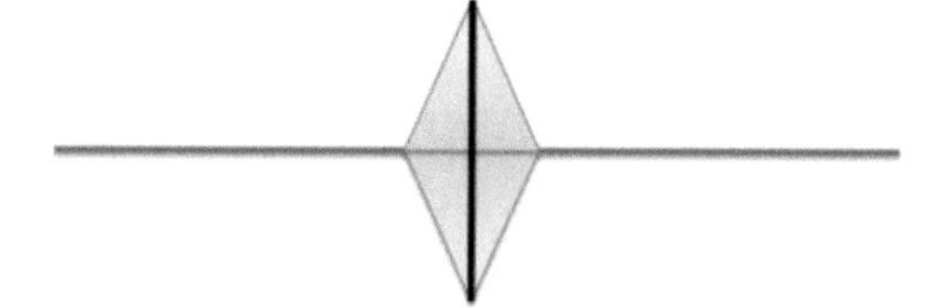

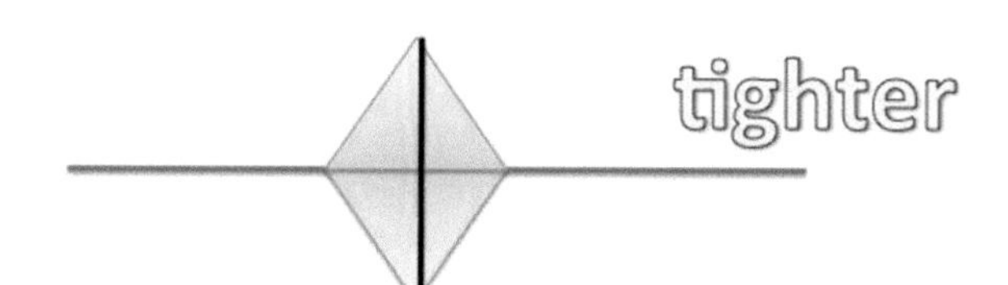

Fig. 9.22 The tighter the suture the greater the spread of the forces on the tissue

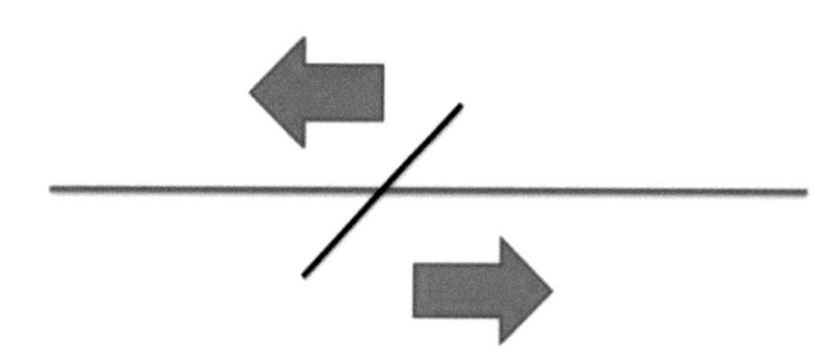

Fig. 9.23 A suture, which is obliquely placed, will create forces which will cause the wound edges to slide and distort the wound

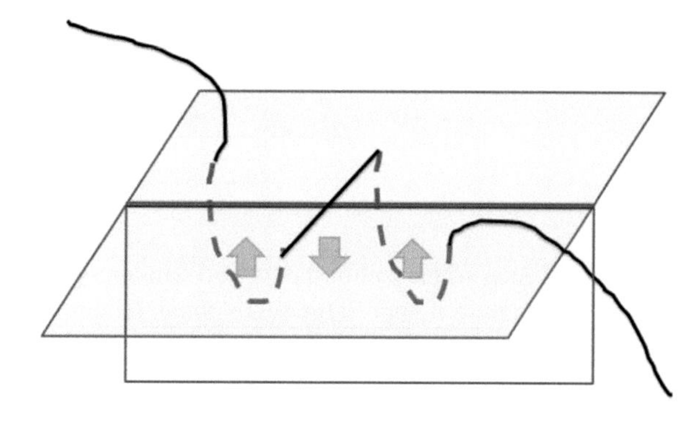

Fig. 9.24 A continuous suture will created forces on the surface and deep within the tissue which may distort the tissue

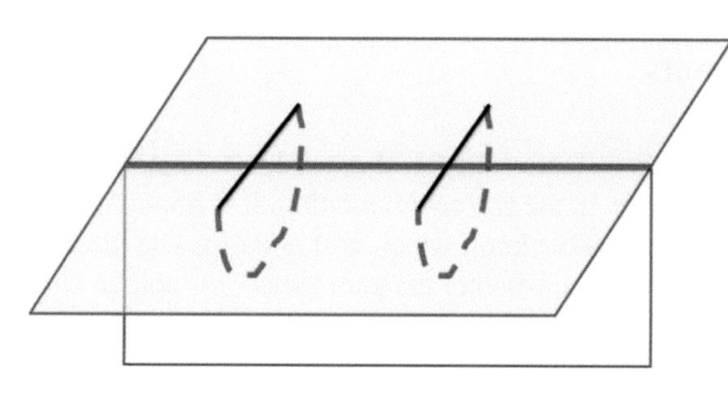

Fig. 9.25 Interrupted sutures exist in one plane and therefore the forces are in line and counter act each other. It is therefore easier to avoid secondary effects

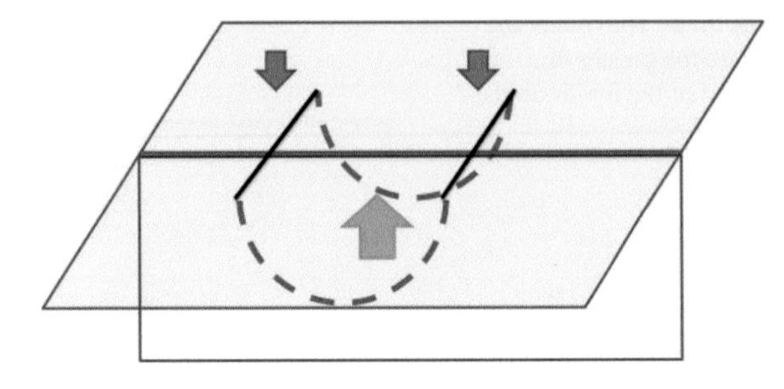

Fig. 9.26 A "mattress" suture will elevate the tissue in the centre

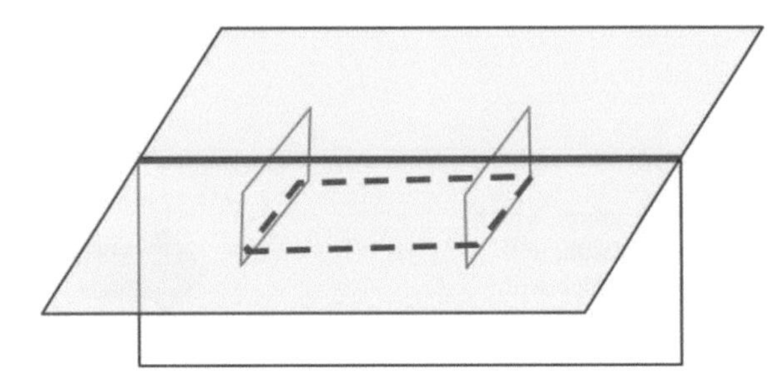

Fig. 9.27 A deep suture on the same plane will hold the tissues together but can be difficult to achieve in thin tissues

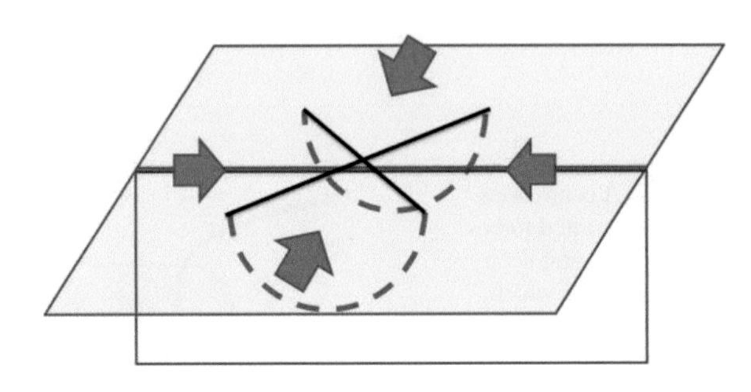

Fig. 9.28 A cross stitch will compress the tissue centrally

A buried deep stitch within the wound can appose the wound with minimal distortion of the suture if kept in the same plane. However the ocular tissues are rarely deep enough to use such a profile. A cross stitch creates tension on the tissue toward the centre of the cross (Figs. 9.27, 9.28 and 9.29).

Knots

The most effective knot is the reef knot. This is achieved by carefully overlapping the sutures in the correct orientation. It is important to create the reef knot profile to achieve a stable knot, which will not slip. The direction of pull on the sutures will also determine whether the knot locks or is able to slip (Figs. 9.30, 9.31, 9.32, 9.33, 9.34, 9.35, 9.36 and 9.37).

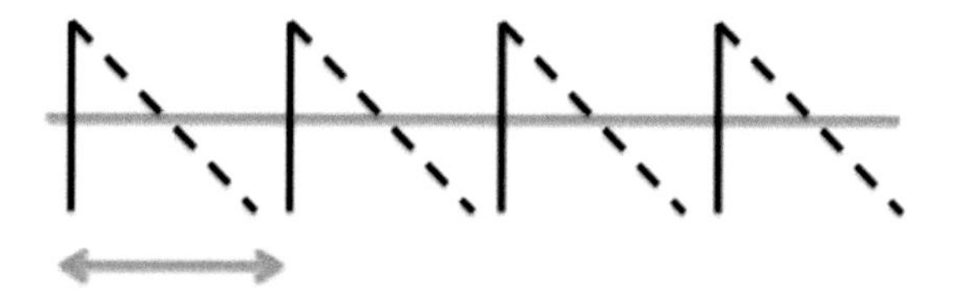

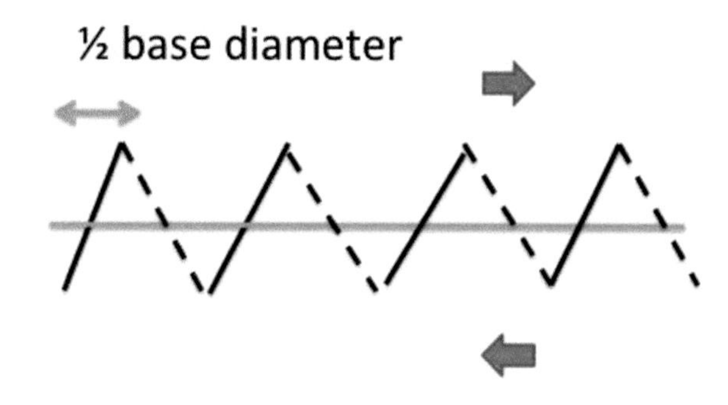

Fig. 9.29 When a single continuous suture is used the suture on tension will want to move the tissue a 1/2 base diameter to take on the second configuration

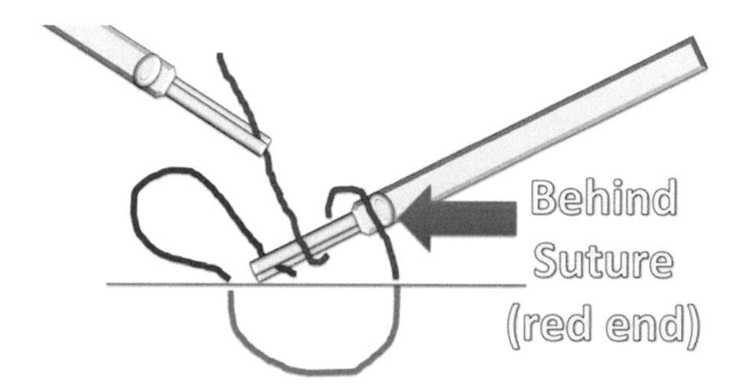

Fig. 9.30 To start a reef knot take the first throw behind the suture as shown

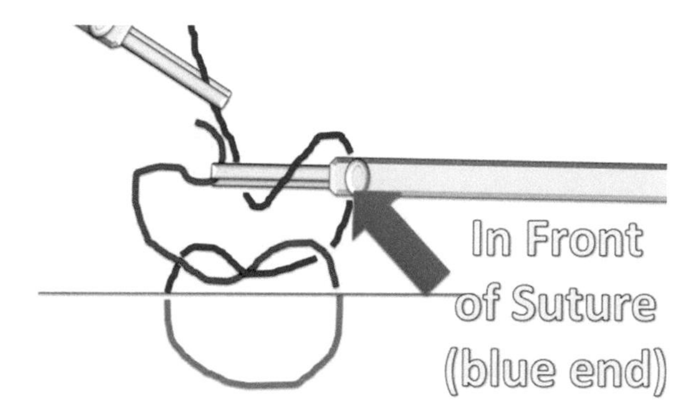

Fig. 9.31 Take the second throw in front of the suture

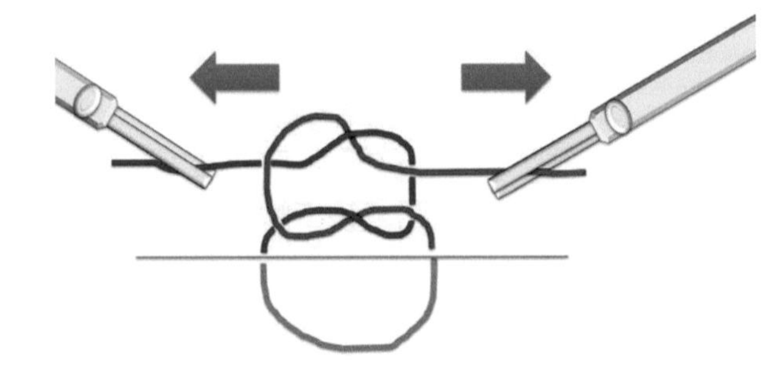

Fig. 9.32 See Fig. 9.31

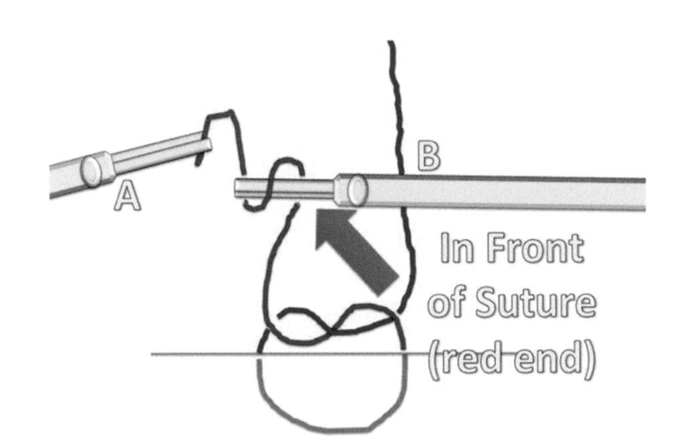

Fig. 9.33 If you do not want to let go of the suture you can make a loop with the instrument in front of the suture at first. Note the forceps A and B switch positions in this sequence

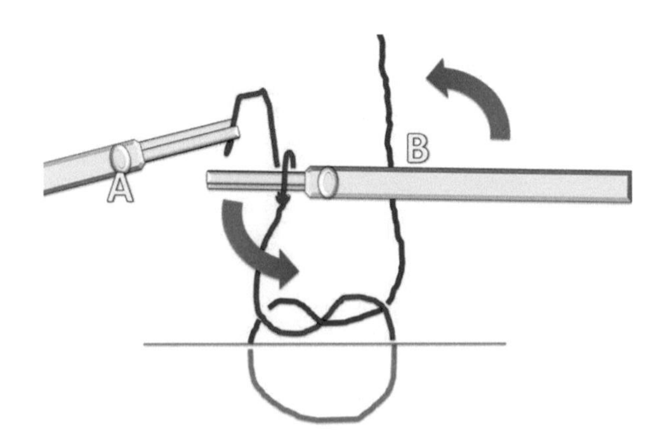

Fig. 9.34 You will need to rotate back on yourself. A and B indicate the forceps

Using the same profile but with increased numbers of overlaps of the suture can also help stabilise the knot. Even asymmetric use of these overlaps of suture can be effective. The asymmetry can be used, once the knot is tightened, to create a shape of knot, which can be easily rotated into the tissue for burying. A knot can be temporarily stabilised by pulling one suture towards the exit site of the suture from the tissue thereby locking it underneath the overlying suture end (Figs. 9.38, 9.39, 9.40, 9.41 and 9.42).

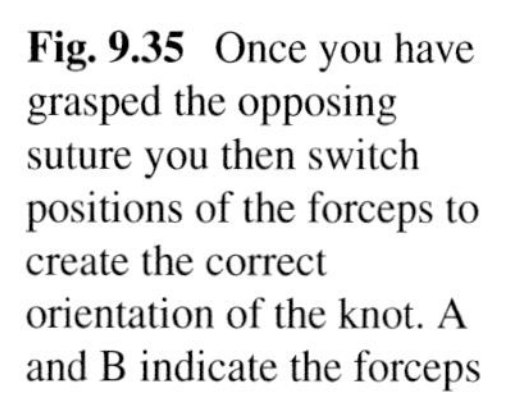

Fig. 9.35 Once you have grasped the opposing suture you then switch positions of the forceps to create the correct orientation of the knot. A and B indicate the forceps

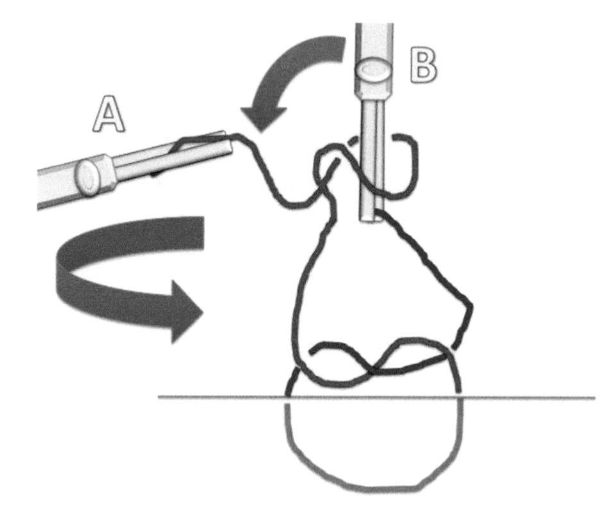

Fig. 9.36 Once the forceps are switched the knot can be tightened. A and B indicate the forceps

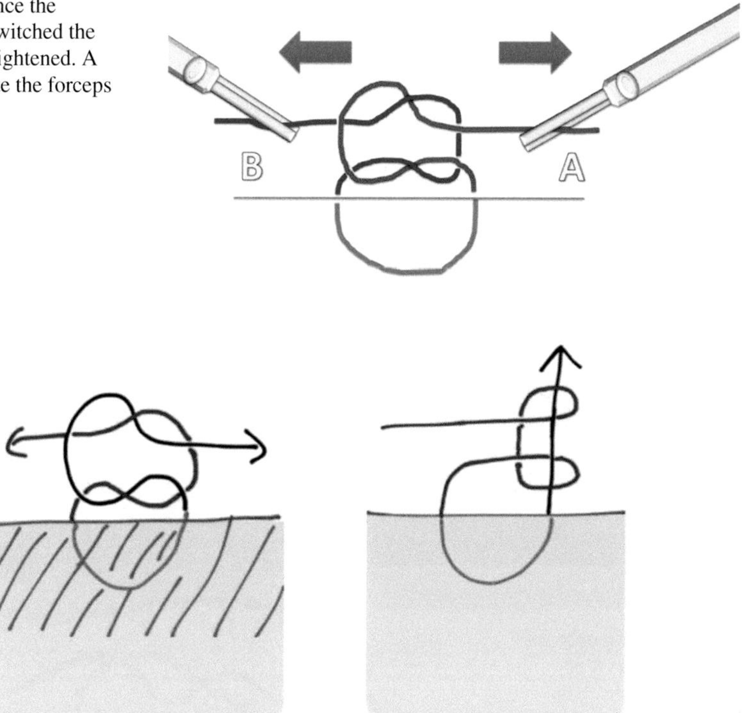

Fig. 9.37 Pulling the sutures horizontally creates a reef knot which will not slip. Pulling one suture vertically creates a slip knot despite the same initial configuration

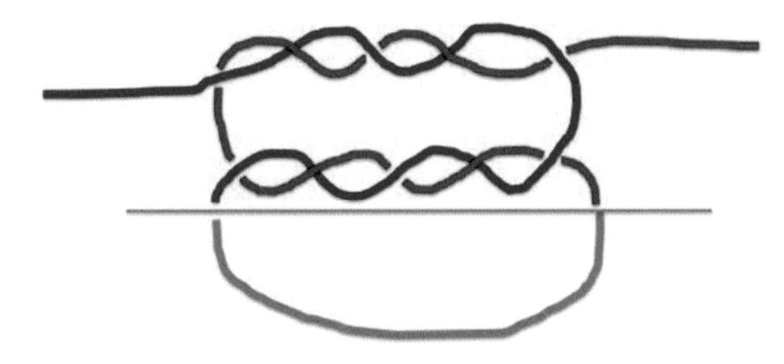

Fig. 9.38 By repeating the reef knot configuration a more secure knot can be created

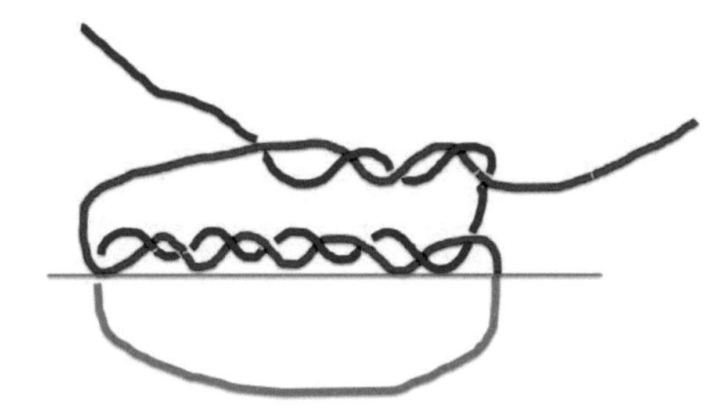

Fig. 9.39 The pattern can be created with different numbers of throws in each layer

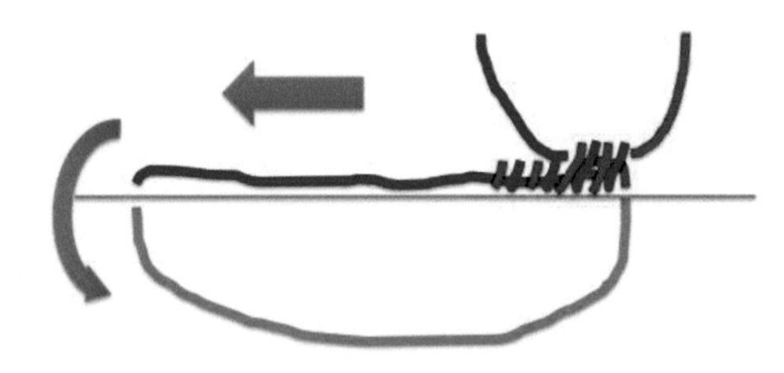

Fig. 9.40 Unequal throws can be used to create an "*arrowhead*" shaped knot which can be easier to bury inside the tissue

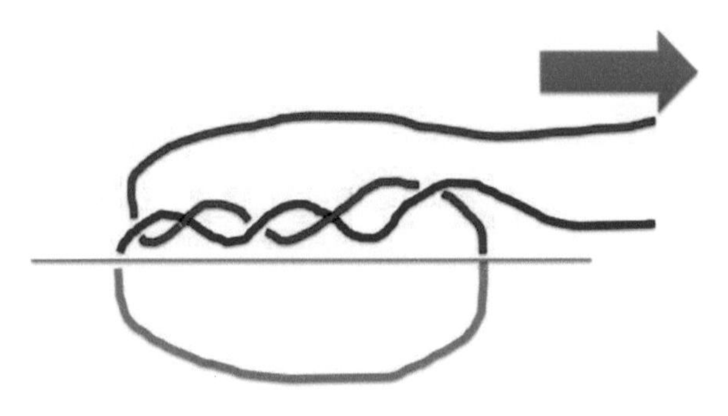

Fig. 9.41 With only one layer of throws it is possible to "*lock*" the sutures to keep tension on the wound temporarily by pulling on one end of the suture dragging it underneath the other suture

Fig. 9.42 The suture is compressed between the second suture end and the tissue preventing slippage

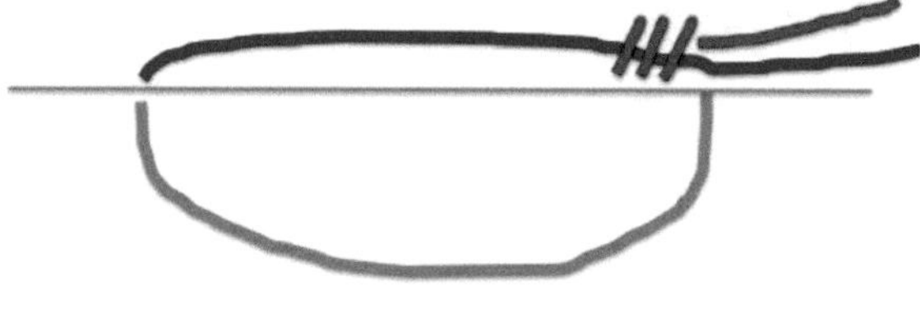

Fig. 9.43 If a knot has been created within the wound to bury it, rotating the knot into the tissue will help stabiles the knot making it more secure, see below

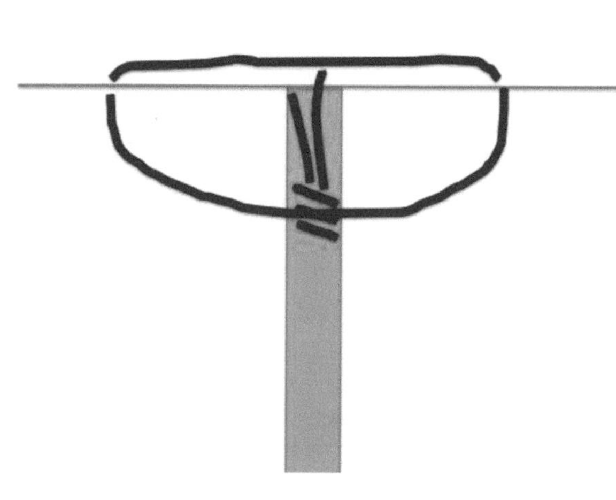

Fig. 9.44 See Fig. 9.43

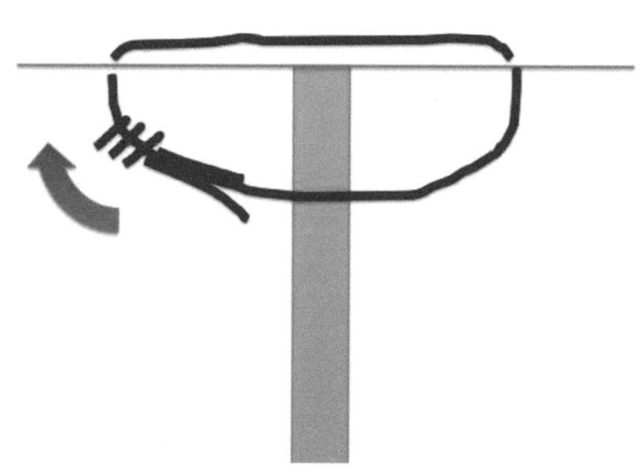

A knot, which has been created within the wound to allow burying, should be drawn into the tissue, this further stabilises the knot preventing it from unraveling (Figs. 9.43, 9.44, 9.45, 9.46, 9.47, 9.48, 9.49, 9.50, 9.51, 9.52, 9.53, 9.54, 9.55 and 9.56)

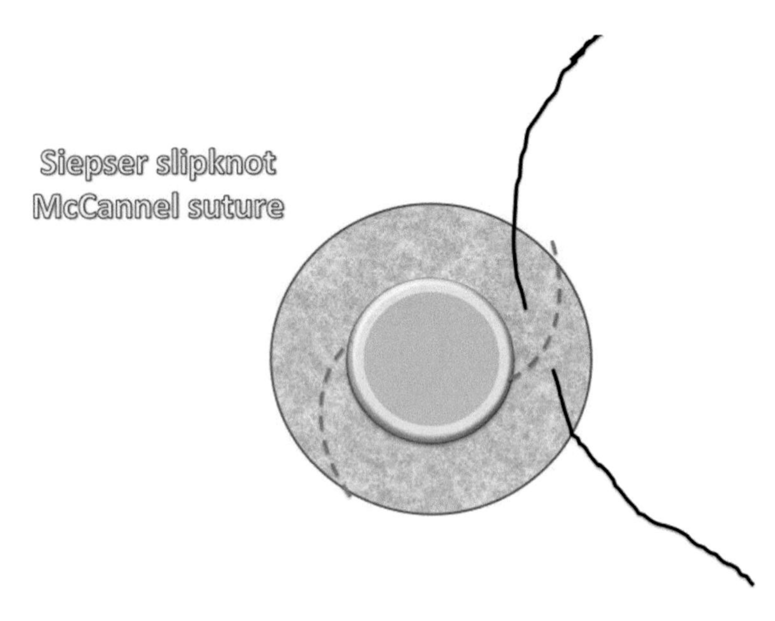

Fig. 9.45 To tie a knot in a confined space use a Siepser knot. For example when tying an IOL to the iris. Insert the suture and exit it through another wound (Chang DF. *J Cataract Refract Surg* 2004; 30:1170–1176)

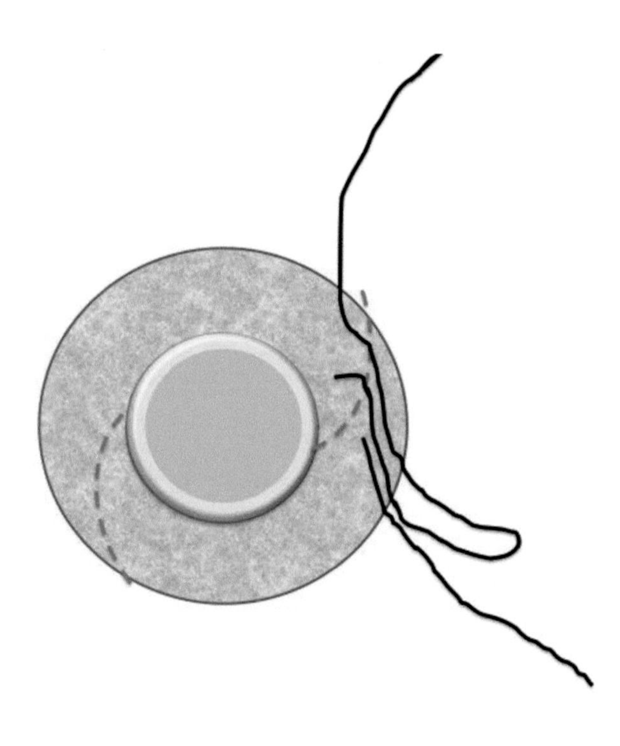

Fig. 9.46 Pull a loop out through the original wound

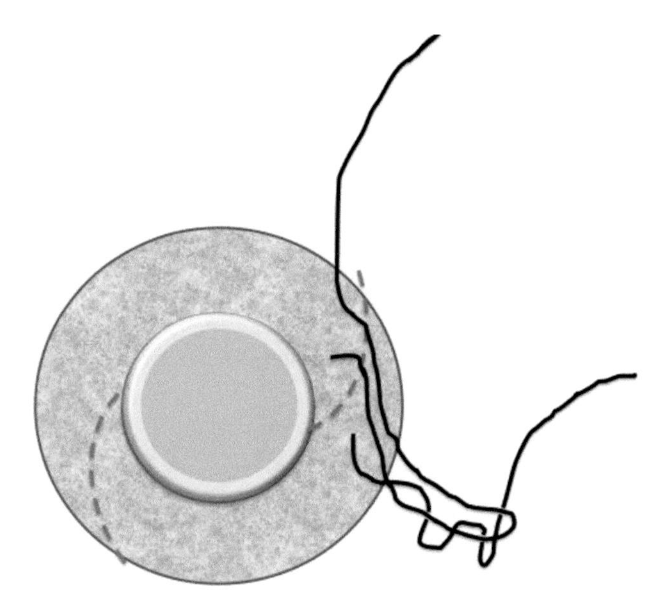

Fig. 9.47 Rotate the free end of the suture through the loop twice

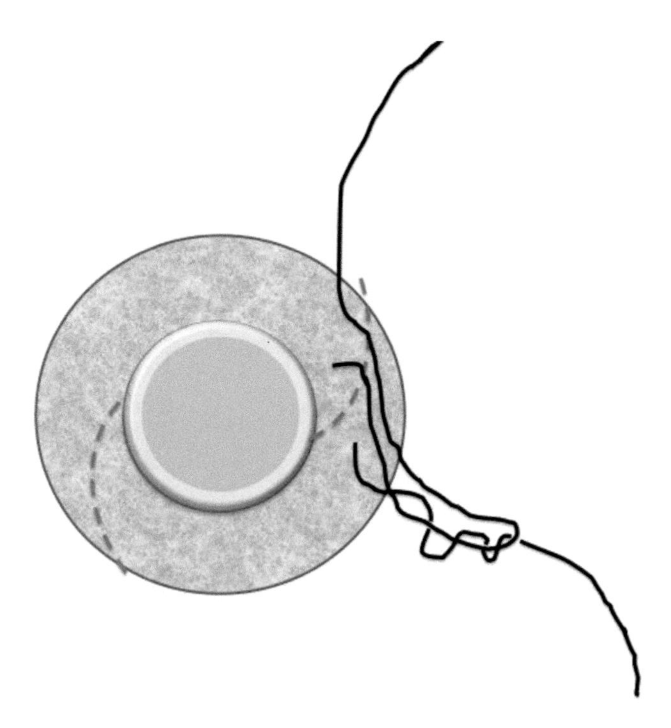

Fig. 9.48 See Fig. 9.47

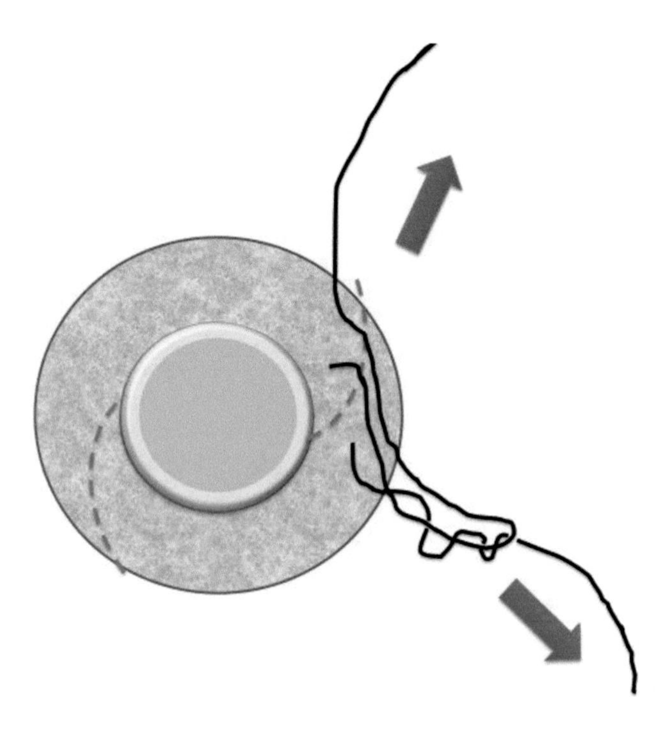

Fig. 9.49 Pull the two free ends

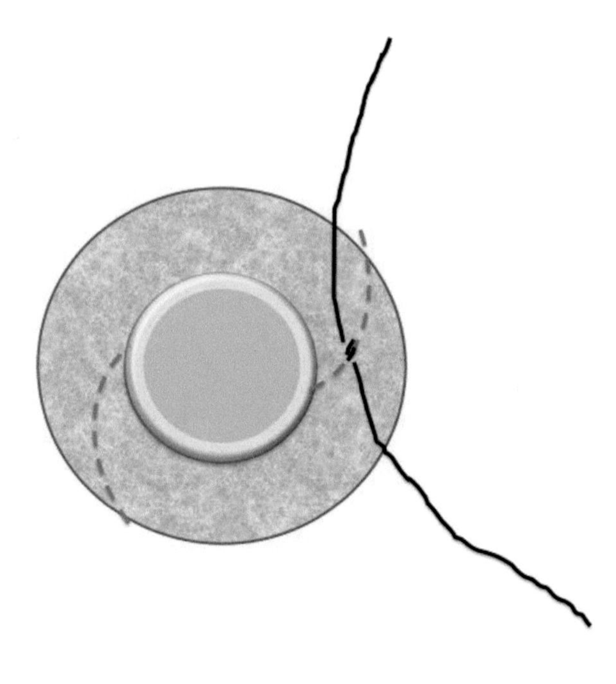

Fig. 9.50 The knot tightens onto the haptic of the IOL

Fig. 9.51 A second throw can be applied to lock the knot

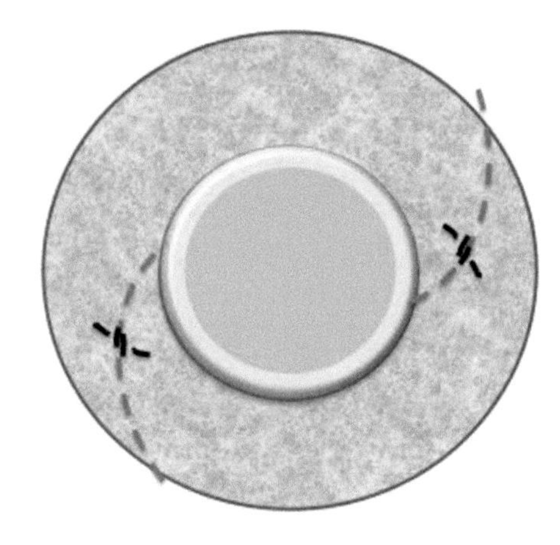

Fig. 9.52 See Fig. 9.51

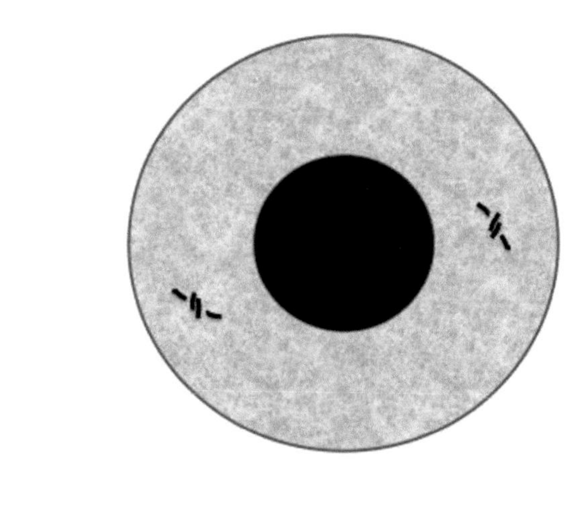

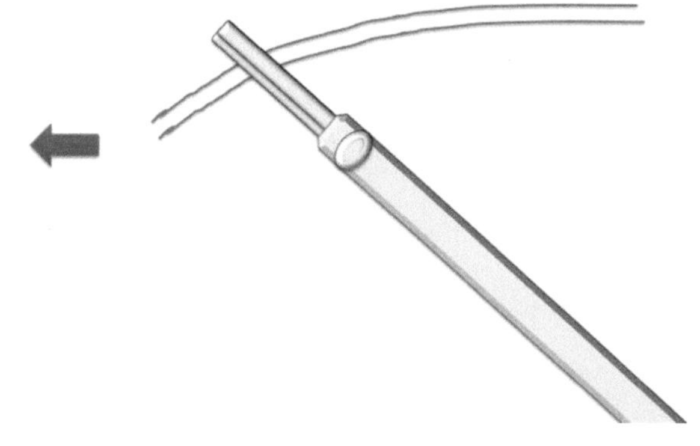

Fig. 9.53 To create a loop in a suture, for example to lock a double suture, use a forcep and create a loop, see below

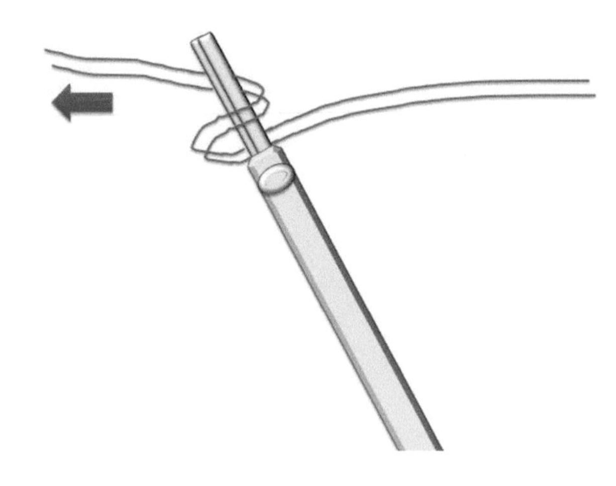

Fig. 9.54 See Fig. 9.53

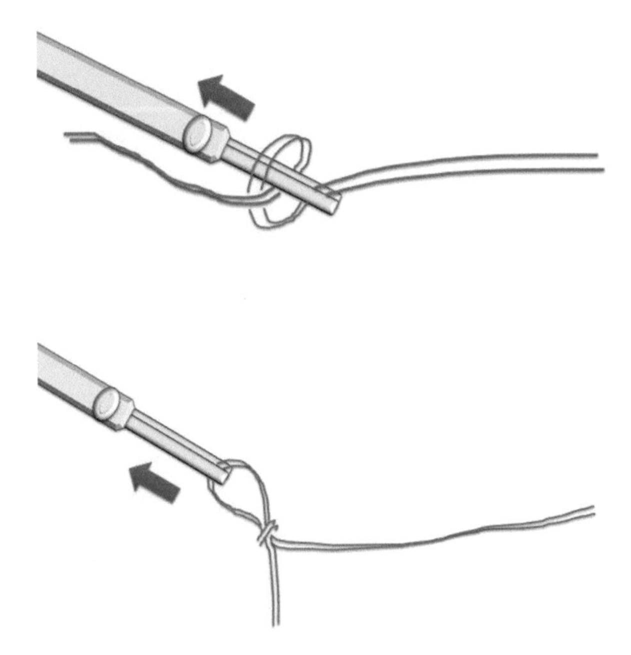

Fig. 9.55 Twist the instrument backwards to pick up the proximal suture

Fig. 9.56 Pull the suture through the loop and tighten

Index

A
Anterior chamber, 73, 77, 80, 87, 90, 105
Anterior segment surgery, 40, 127
Arc of safety, 95, 97–109
Argon lasers, 136–138
Aspiration, 116, 121, 129
  of fluid, 112
  fluid flow, 115
  procedures, 105

B
Balanced salt solution in water (BSS), 125
Bancroft rule, 132
Bernoulli's Principle, 115–118, 125
Boyle's law, 133
Broad blade, 44
Bulk modulus, 12, 13

C
CCC. *See* Continuous curvilinear capsulorhexis (CCC)
Choroidal haemorrhage
  extra-capsular cataract extraction, 92
  finite element analysis, 93, 96
  globe distortion, 93–94
  incidence, 92
  instrument
    adjustment on, 97–100
    arc of safety, 95, 97–104
    compensatory retraction, 98
    J-shaped movement, 99, 105
    movement, restriction of, 99
    obstructions to movement of, 105, 106
    overlap arcs of safety, 105, 108–109
    safe movement, 98
  ocular hypotony, 92
  suprachoroidal space, 92
Clear corneal zone, 49, 50
Continuous curvilinear capsulorhexis (CCC), 62–68
  and capsular fold configurations
    double fold configuration, 73, 79
    single fold configuration, 72
    zero fold configuration, 71
  size
    and nucleus cracking, 76
    and nucleus rotation, 73
  Young's modulus of lens, 68–70
Continuous suture, 148–153, 155
Curved wound, 43, 46, 48, 52, 149
Cystotome, 72

D
Darcy's law, 131
Density, 10, 13, 15
Diode lasers, 138, 140, 141
Diode pumped solid-state lasers, 138
Double fold configuration, 73, 79
Double frequency YAG lasers, 138, 139
Dye lasers, 138

E
80/20 rule. *See* Pereto principle
Emulsion, 132

T.H. Williamson, *Intraocular Surgery: A Basic Surgical Guide*,
DOI 10.1007/978-3-319-27990-9

Evaporation
  incompressible during surgery, 132–133
  Pascal's Principle, 133
  vapour pressure, 132
Excimer laser, 137
Extrude and Revolve techniques, 15

F
Fibre optic instruments, 136
Fick's Diffusion equation, 133
Filters, 135
Finite element analysis (FEA), ophthalmology
  material properties
    application of force, 10
    Bulk modulus, 12, 13
    density, 13, 15
    for ocular tissues, 10
    Poisson ratio, 13, 14
    Shear modulus, 12–13
    Young's modulus of elasticity and yield strength, 10, 12
  meshed model, 16, 17
  microsurgical procedures, 49
  surgical planes
    continuous curvilinear capsulorhexis (*see* Continuous curvilinear capsulorhexis (CCC))
    and corneal section, 49–62
    in microsurgery, 49
    nucleus cracking into quadrants, 78, 80, 82–86
    nucleus rotation, 78, 81
    sculpting central groove, 76, 81
  tissue geometry, 15–16
Flow
  of fluid, 112, 114, 115
    Bernoulli's Principle, 125
    Hagan Poiseuille Law, 126
    Laplace's Law, 126
    Reynold's Number, 126–127
  rate, 112–113, 123, 125
  of tissue, 116
  velocity, 116
Fluids
  balanced salt solution in water, 125
  Bernoulli's Principle, 125
  convection, Darcy's law, 131
  diffusion
    Fick's law, 130
    Stokes Einstein, 131
  emulsion, 132
  evaporation
    incompressible during surgery, 132–133
    Pascal's Principle, 133
    vapour pressure, 132
  flow rate, 125
  gases
    Boyle's law, 133
    Fick's diffusion equation, 133
    molecules separation, 134
    surface tension, 133
  Hagan Poiseuille Law, 126
  injecting into eye, 126–127
  interfacial tension between two liquids, 132
  Laplace's Law for pressure, 126
  outflow, 87
  Reynold's Number, 126
  viscoelastic fluids, 127, 129–131
  viscosity, 127–129
Forceps
  angle, 22
  blind spot, 27–29
  capsulorhexis, 68, 77
  intraocular, 68
  with platform, 25
  round and sharp edged, 21, 23, 24
  serrated, 31–32
  simple, 25
  toothed, 21, 57

G
Gases
  Boyle's law, 133
  compressible, 133
  Fick's diffusion equation, 133
  molecules separation, 134
  surface tension, 133
Guillotine cutters, 111, 116–118, 121–123

H
Hagan Poiseuille Law, 111–112, 126
Hypotony, 6, 92

I
Incisions
  by action of instrumentation, 42
  circular, 59
  flat, 55
  length, 49, 57–58

oblique, 51
perpendicular, 51, 54, 55
variation, 43
Instruments
action of scissors, 28
angulation of, 28, 34–38
effectiveness of, 25–26
forceps
angle, 22
blind spot, 27–29
with platform, 25
round and sharp edged, 21, 23, 24
serrated, 31–32
simple, 25
toothed, 21
function, 21
size, 28
Interfacial tension, 132
Intraocular pressure, 39, 93, 94, 96, 111
Iris, 9, 13, 49, 50, 115, 116, 141, 160

K
Keratome, 49, 50
Knots
reef knot
"arrowhead" shaped, 158
burying into tissue, 159–160
numbers of throws, 158
pull direction, 154–157
repeating configuration, 158
Siepser knot, 160–164

L
Laplace's Law, 126
Laser
absorption of wavelengths, 139, 141
application, 138, 140–141
argon, 136–138
diode lasers, 140, 141
excimer, 137
Nd:YAG laser, 137, 141
per-operatively via fibre-optic instruments, 140–141
photon, 139
thermal burn, 139
thermal effect, 139, 140
yellow lasers, 139
Lens
capsule, 87, 90, 99, 104
vs. lens cortex, 68, 77
CCC, 76
multifocal, 62
obstruction to instruments movement, 106
phacoemulsification, 116, 117
sculpting central groove, 76, 81, 84–86
shear distribution on, 78, 82
Light
field of view, 135
intensity, 139
sources, 135
Light amplification by stimulated emission of radiation. *See* Laser
Liquid, 9, 95, 112
flow, 125–127
incompressible during surgery, 132–133
interfacial tension, 132
intermolecular attractions in, 134
vapour pressure, 132
viscoelastic, 127, 129–130
viscosity, 127–129

M
Machines
and eye, fluid flow between
Bernoulli's principle, 115–118
flow rate, 112–114
Hagan Poiseuille Law, 111–112
infusion heights, 114
pars plana vitrectomy, 111
phacoemulsification
devices, 111
lateral motion, 119
mechanism, 118
tip, 115–116
Margin of safety, 2
Mattress sutures, 151, 154
Micro forceps, 143
Microscopes, 27, 49, 50, 76, 81, 135

N
Narrow blade, 44
Needle, 51
phaco, 118
round bodied, 55, 62
of suture track, 144–145
wound distortion, 144
Neodymium:yttrium-aluminum-garnet (Nd:YAG) laser, 137, 141
Non-Newtonian properties, 127
Nucleus cracking, and capsulorhexis size, 76, 80
Nucleus rotation, and capsulorhexis size, 73

O

Oblique wounds, 146
Oval shaped capsulotomies, 62

P

Pascal's principle, 133
Pereto principle, 6–7
Perfluorocarbons, 132
Perfluoropropane, 133
Peristaltic pump, 114
Phaco
  time, 119
  tip deeper, 100
Phacoemulsification
  devices, 111
  lateral motion, 119
  mechanism, 118
  power, 118–119
  tip, 115–116
  ultrasonic cutters, 118
  zone interactions, 118
Photocoagulation, 139
Piezo electric crystals, 111
Poisson effect, 13
Poisson ratio, 13, 14, 23

Q

Q-switch mode, 141

R

Ragged wound, 149, 151
Reef knots
  "arrowhead" shaped, 158
  burying into tissue, 159–160
  different throws, 156, 158
  pulling direction, 154–157
  repeating configuration, 156, 158
  unequal throws, 156, 158
Retinal detachment, 89–91
Reynold's Number, 126

S

Scissors, 28, 45, 50–51, 53, 54, 71
Sclera, 9, 12, 13, 49, 52, 57, 58, 89, 93
Shear modulus, 12–13
Shear stress, 13, 14, 73, 76, 78, 80, 82–86, 93, 96, 127
Shelved wound, 146, 148
Silicone oil, 126, 132
Single fold configuration, 72
Sophisticated ophthalmic machines, 18
Stepped wound, 146, 147
Strain force, 10
Stress force, 10
Suprachoroidal space, 92
Surface tension, 133
Surgical compartments
  choroidal haemorrhage
    extra-capsular cataract extraction, 92
    FEA zonular support, 100, 105
    finite element analysis, 93, 96
    globe distortion, 93–94
    incidence, 92
    instrument adjustment, 97–100
    ocular hypotony, 92
    suprachoroidal space, 92
  pressure on
    infusion involvement, 87, 89, 91–93
    maintaining, 91, 95
    membrane distortion, 92
    movement of membrane, 89, 94
    nucleus of lens, 87, 90
Surgical drift, 6
Surgical methods and outcomes
  changing methods, 2, 4, 5
  clinical outcomes, 1
  compartmentalization, 7
  complications, 5
  early majority, 7
  environmental factor, 7–8
  margin of safety, 2
  Pereto principle, 6–7
  reduce error, 7
  risks and benefits, 2, 3
  simplification, 7
  surgical drift, 6
Sutures
  buried deep stitch, 154
  compression, 152
  continuous, 148–153, 155
  cross stitch, 154
  holding procedure, 143
  inserting, 147–148
  interrupted, 149, 151, 153
  knots
    overlapping orientation, 154
    reef knot (*see* Reef knots)
    Siepser knot, 160–164
  mattress, 151, 154
  oblique wound risks, 146–147
  over tightening, 145–146
  placement, 149, 152–153
  restoring wound's integrity, 146–149
  semicircular suture track profile, 144
  tension, 146, 154, 155
  track, 144–145
  zigzag, 148, 150

T
Thermal zone, 118
Tissue geometry, 15–16
Torsional motion, 119
Trabeculectomy, 52
Triangular blade, 43, 46
Triangulated wounds, 149

U
Ultrasonic transducer, 111

V
Vacuum, 114
Vapour pressure, 132
Viscoelastic fluids, 127, 129–131
Viscosity, 127–129
Visualisation, 21, 27, 30, 31, 49, 105, 135
Vitrectomy, 114
  compartments, 7
  cutters, 123
  devices, 111
Vitreous cavity, 106

W
Wound
  chevron shaped, 39, 41
  curved, 43, 46, 48, 51
  diagonal, 40
  incisions by instrumentation
    broad blade, 43, 44
    conjunctiva, 48
    mobile tissue, 43, 45, 47
    narrow blade, 42, 44
    symmetrical blade, 48
    triangular blade, 43, 46
  partially sloped, 41
  perpendicular, 39, 41
  self-sealing, 57
  shelved, 40
  short, 66, 67
  sloped, 39, 42
  S-shaped, 50, 53
  stiff and soft tissue, 39
  3-D profile, 40
  vertical perpendicular, 40
  width and length, 42
Wound closure, 144
Wound distorting, 145

Y
Yag laser, 141
Yellow lasers, 139
Young's modulus, 10, 12, 23

Z
Zero fold configuration, 71